WHY YOU DON'T

The most comprehensive appra
facts and figures involved in the

Margaret & Mike
Christmas   '86

WHY YOU DON'T NEED MEAT

PETER COX

THORSONS PUBLISHING GROUP
Wellingborough · New York

First published 1986

© PETER COX 1986

British Library Cataloguing in Publication Data

Cox, Peter
    Why you don't need meat.
    1. Diet
    I. Title
    613.2   RA784

    ISBN 0-7225-1298-8

Printed and bound in Great Britain

Contents

DEDICATION

*This book is dedicated to
all people with open minds*

Acknowledgements

Writing and researching this book has been a very happy experience. Many kind people have helped me and taken an extraordinary interest in the project. My greatest debt of gratitude goes to Peggy, who has worked alongside me throughout, up at all unearthly hours of the day and night as we collected our evidence from computer databases all over the world. I also want to thank the staff of all the libraries I have used, particularly Mrs M. E. Moore of the Sir Thomas Browne Library, and the staff at Addenbrookes Hospital Library, Cambridge. It is unfortunate that so many people who have helped me must remain unidentified at their own request, but to those people working in governmental organizations, the veterinary profession and the food industry I wish to express a very special gratitude, for helping to put me on the right track, at no small risk to themselves. Finally, I would like to mention all the friends I made while working for four very brief months as the first Chief Executive of the Vegetarian Society of the United Kingdom, and thank them for their continuing help and encouragement. This book is a fulfilment of the promises I made them.

PETER COX

Introduction

Every year in this country the meat industry spends a staggering sum of money — running into countless millions of pounds — trying to ensure that you keep on eating meat.

Imagine yourself going out onto every street of every city, town and village in the land and giving a pound away to each man, woman and child you met — on the condition that they promised to carry on buying meat. Well, *that's* the amount of money the meat industry spends in one year just to keep the consumer wanting its products.

Put like that, it may sound like bribery.

Personally, I believe it is. Because what we're talking about is intensive, high-pressure advertising. The sort you — and your children — can't escape from. You see it everywhere, all the time — on television, on posters, at the cinema, on the radio, in the newspapers . . .

When I worked in the advertising business we'd call it 'saturation coverage'. The consumer can't help being exposed to it — time and time and time again. Eventually, the message gets through — rather like brainwashing. And it *does* work. Believe me, they wouldn't spend one penny of their precious advertising budgets *unless* they were going to get a very, very good return indeed.

They can afford to spend such large sums of money because the size of the meat industry is absolutely staggering. When you add it all up, it runs into *thousands of millions of pounds* every year. So in comparison, the millions they spend on promotion is really quite small — almost chicken feed, in fact.

The meat industry spends that money on advertising with only one objective. To ensure that their consumers — and that means *you* — keep on buying meat. Quite simply, they can't afford to let you *stop* buying it, or even to allow you to cut back on the quantity you buy. And they will do virtually anything they can to prevent you from changing your buying habits.

But even the meat industry can't fool all of the people all of the time. Incredibly, things *are* starting to change. More and more quite ordinary people are beginning to wonder whether they're being taken for a ride. For one thing, many people are starting to feel genuinely worried about the quality of food they're buying. The major supermarkets know this, and they haven't been slow to catch on. They're starting to exert pressure on their suppliers to produce better food and healthier food: food which is *really* fit for human consumption. It's about time.

And something else is happening, too. A revolution is taking place in the high street. Butchers' shops are starting to close down and disappear; some of them are changing into delicatessens, some of them are even starting to sell fresh fruit and vegetables. 'If you can't beat them,' said one butcher recently as he put a selection of meat-free meals on sale in his shop, 'you've got to join them.'[1] And even their own trade journal has recently labelled the butcher an 'endangered species', while calling for swift action to stop him disappearing completely. The meat trade is getting frightened, too. Recently, an order went out from the very top to ban any public debates with its critics. 'We would be wasting our time,' pronounced a director of the Meat Promotion Executive, 'if we entered into a slanging match, *which we could only lose.*'[2]

Yes, a quiet revolution is taking place, the like of which we've never seen before. But don't expect to hear, read or see much about it in the media. Because there are no multi-million pound advertising budgets available to put the case *against* eating meat — there's no profit in it. In fact, I predict that over the next few years the meat trade will be spending even more money on advertising and promotion, in a tougher and tougher battle to persuade you to go on buying their products. It looks very much as if the consumer is in for a very hard sell indeed. In the business, we used to call it 'defensive marketing', and it's the very hardest thing to undertake. When people go off your product in a big way, it's almost impossible to persuade them to change their minds.

So what exactly *is* happening out there in the marketplace? I can give you some independent figures, produced by a well-known market research firm, that may shed some light on the picture.[3]

According to this research, there are in this country at the present time well over *three million people* who have completely cut out meat from their diets. The remarkable thing is that this figure has grown by a staggering thirty per cent in just twelve months. That in itself is enough to indicate that something pretty profound is happening. But there's more. Seventeen million people in this country have reduced their consumption of meat to some extent in the past year. That's one person in every three. Perhaps you can now see why the meat industry is very, very worried. Because the total drop in meat consumption may only be small at the moment, but what if it's the tip of the iceberg . . ?

So why are more and more people cutting down on the meat they eat? I think I can explain by telling you a story about a family I know. I want to call it Joe's Story, because he's twelve years old and the youngest son, and deserves all the credit.

One day, Joe came home from school. He had a problem, and his mother, Susan, could see it written all over his young face.

'Are you going to tell me what's worrying you?', she asked him.

Joe frowned, and didn't answer directly. Instead he asked his mother a question.

'Mum, what's for tea?'

'Beans on toast. Is that all right for you?'

'Yes,' said Joe. 'That's all right. But I don't think I want to eat any more meat. I don't think I like it any more.'

His mother listened. Joe didn't fuss over his food, he usually ate what he was given, unless he was ill. And he didn't look ill.

'What's bothering you about it, Joe?' she asked.

'Meat is dead animals, isn't it?' said Joe. 'We talked about it in school today. A butcher came and talked to all of us, and I told him I didn't like killing animals.'

Susan knew what Joe meant, because it had troubled her too when she had been a child. But she'd done nothing about it, because her parents would have been alarmed if their daughter had suddenly stopped eating meat. She didn't talk any more about it then, but discussed it with her husband that evening. They agreed to let Joe eat what he wanted for a couple of days, but if it lasted any longer, then Susan would have to talk it over with their doctor. And so, a few days later, she found herself in the doctor's surgery.

'Don't worry about it,' he advised her. 'I'd prefer Joe to stop eating hamburgers rather than to stop eating fresh vegetables. He's growing, but he can get all the nourishment he needs from a meat-free diet.'

'But what about his protein?' Susan asked. 'He needs lots of protein, where else can he get it from?'

The doctor smiled. 'You know, most of the diseases we suffer from in the West are diseases of affluence — too many calories, too much fat, not enough exercise. We do have a nutritional problem, but it's a problem of excess nutrition rather than malnutrition. For a boy Joe's age, the minimum recommended protein intake is about 50 grams a day — that's just under two ounces. It's not difficult to get that. A couple of ounces of Cheddar cheese, three or four slices of bread, and maybe a cereal dish like macaroni, for instance — a glass of milk (skimmed, preferably) and you've covered the basic requirements. Do you think you can manage that?'

'Oh yes, that's no problem. But I still feel totally ignorant about his other nutritional needs, like vitamins, and so on. What can I do about that?'

'Well,' said the doctor, 'there's no easy answer to that. In fact, very few people actually know what their body's requirements are. I believe they're starting to include it with health education in some schools, but that won't help *you*. But it's often only when people change their diets, like your Joe is doing, that they actually begin to be aware of what they're eating. Far too many people still go through life without giving a moment's thought to their diet. So you could see this as a sort of opportunity. All I can say is, eat as varied a diet as possible, include lots of fresh food, especially green leafy vegetables, read some books and pick up some of the free leaflets that are around, such as the Health Education Council's. All right?'

Susan still felt rather worried, but there was not much else she could ask. As she was leaving, her doctor made a final remark:

'You know, both you and your husband could do a lot worse than follow Joe's example. It can be a very healthy way of living.'

All this happened a year ago. Today, Joe is doing very nicely without meat, and Susan is feeling much happier about it. It became increasingly difficult to provide two sets of meals in the house — one with meat, and one without, so the rest of the household found that they, too, were eating more and more meals without meat. Eventually, Susan gave it up completely, and her husband hardly eats it either — although he'll sometimes choose fish if they're eating out. Their lives have changed, in a good way, and they all say they feel healthier and more alive than they did. And it's all due to Joe.

This is a pattern that is being repeated all the time, all over the country. But it's not *just* young people who are turning away from meat. Old people — in their seventh or even eighth decades — are changing a lifetime's habit, and reporting positive health benefits. Many say their arthritis disappears. Rheumatic and aching joints are eased. People chronically ill, some with cancer, are experimenting with a fresh food diet, and getting physical and spiritual renewal from it. Other people — those who are concerned about our world and our environment — are also acting in a personal way to try and bring about positive change. After all, meat is a terribly wasteful commodity. For every one hundred pounds of plant protein that we feed to cows (soya beans and other animal feed), only *five pounds* of it is converted into meat. The rest — ninety-five pounds — is turned into slurry. What a criminal waste of basic food in a hungry world.

All over the country, more and more people are thinking the same way. They are asserting their right *not* to do what the giants of the meat industry want them to do. And they are finding that their new lifestyle really suits them down to the ground.

But even so, most people still don't know the complete story. They don't know the full horror of an industry that puts profit before health and morality. They don't realise the overwhelming weight of evidence that now exists *against* meat — evidence that I've pieced together from all over the world, and which has never before been assembled and made public in such a comprehensive way.

The meat industry spends millions of pounds every year trying to persuade you to buy their products. This book puts the other side of the case — the side they *don't* want you to know about.

REFERENCES

1.   *Meat Trades Journal*, 5 September 1985.
2.   *Meat Trades Journal*, 13 June 1985.
3.   Gallup Poll, commissioned by The Realeat Co.

1

Connections

It must have been one of those days. The two doctors had got into the hospital lift, pressed their floor buttons, and then stood in the slightly awkward silence that usually prevails inside lifts for a few seconds until the doors open and the passengers are free to leave. But this time, the doors didn't open.

'I just don't believe it!', said one of them. 'This happened to me last week. It took half an hour to get out.'

The other doctor was busy pushing every button in sight. 'We'd better get on the emergency phone,' he said. 'I can't make any of these buttons work.'

While help was on its way, they chatted about patients and cases and other medical subjects, in the abstract way that doctors do. As luck would have it — extremely good luck, as it turned out — one of them happened to be a paediatrician, and the other was a gynaecologist.

'You know,' said the paediatrician, 'I'm seeing more cases of vaginal cancer in young girls than I've ever seen before. It makes me think that there must be some sort of common factor to it. Nothing I can track it down to, though.'

'Really?', said the gynaecologist. Just at that moment, he was more interested in getting out of the lift than in listening to his colleague's case notes. He paused, and thought about the words he had just heard. 'I suppose you've checked on their mothers' medical history, have you?'

'Oh yes', said the other. 'But there doesn't seem to be much there. These girls are all going through puberty. I can't imagine that anything their mothers would have done ten to fifteen years ago could make much difference now. Although' — here he grew thoughtful — 'most of them *were* difficult pregnancies. I think quite a lot of them took stilboestrol'. He looked at the gynaecologist. 'What do you know about it?'

The gynaecologist thought for a moment.

'It's an artificial hormone', he said. 'I'm sure it's safe. There's been at least one study about it. We used to prescribe stilboestrol for certain complications, but the thinking nowadays is that it doesn't seem to make much difference, except to make the pregnancy a bit longer'.

There were sounds from outside. A widening chink of light started to appear through the doors, and the two men prepared to leave their temporary prison.

'I tell you what', said the gynaecologist. 'I'll check into it for you. Why don't you give me a call in a day or two?' And with that, the doors opened, and they left.

A few days later the two doctors met up again. The drug — diethyl stilboestrol — was now their main topic of conversation, and they were both very excited about the pattern they could see emerging. They found that diethyl stilboestrol (or DES, for short) had been prescribed to women ever since a paper published in an American gynaecological journal had recommended it to prevent repeated reproductive failures and other complications of pregnancy. They found that a clinical trial of the artificial hormone, involving some 2000 women from 1950 to 1952, had concluded that it had no effect on pregnancies, except to prolong them a little. But there was no mention of any side-effects.[1]

There had been no further trials since then. It was assumed by everyone in the medical field that, although DES probably didn't help difficult pregnancies, it probably didn't do any harm either. So clinicians still continued to use it if they felt it might be useful for a woman. For example, at the famous Mayo clinic, in Rochester, Minnesota, about ten per cent of all pregnant women were given

DES between 1946 and 1951. And during the 1960s about 25,000 women in total received the drug in the United States. Then, in 1971, the evidence started to fit together.

A previously rare cancer, clear-cell adenocarcinoma, began to be seen with increasing frequency in young women who had been born between 1946 and 1951, *and whose mothers had been given* DES. Then other, non-cancerous changes in the genital tracts of other young girls began to be reported, too. And finally, it was also proven that tumorous effects could even be traced in the *sons* of women who had been treated with the hormone. Cases of prostate cancer, male bladder cancer and cancer of the testicles were diagnosed and positively associated with DES. The evidence was now absolutely conclusive. DES could cause cancer and a variety of other diseases in the children of women who had been unlucky enough to be dosed. But it didn't necessarily show up for years — sometimes in children as young as seven, but sometimes not until the mid or late twenties. For the poor children, it was a silent time bomb, ticking away for years, until something (often puberty) happened to make it go off.[2]

Perhaps the saddest and cruellest part of the DES disaster is that a new analysis of old data now clearly shows that DES *did* have an effect on pregnant women. They had more abortions, neonatal deaths and premature births than they would otherwise have had.

It is estimated that about two million women were treated with DES before the full facts were known. But, at least, we'd learnt something, hadn't we? Now medical science could prove that DES was a disaster, and shouldn't come anywhere near a pregnant woman. It would never happen again, would it?

'Never' is a final, absolute word. And where human greed is concerned, there are no absolutes. Some people will always want just a little bit more, regardless of the cost in suffering or human life itself. We hadn't heard the last of DES.

The Meat Connection

From the meat producer's point of view, the attraction of DES as a drug is that it is a terrifically powerful growth promoter — it can make any animal put on weight incredibly quickly. And more weight equals more profit. Now, meat producers have been experimenting with altering the balance of sex hormones in their animals for a long time. They have been willing to try *anything* that tips the scales in their favour when the slaughtered animal's carcass is weighed in the abattoir. One very old way of doing this has been to castrate male animals. Another extremely widespread practice is to make a cow pregnant about two months before she is slaughtered. Of course, the baby calf dies in its mother's womb before it's born, but it's all valuable extra weight. Then they discovered DES . . .

We pick up the thread of the next connection in a doctor's surgery in Milan, in early 1978. An Italian woman sits in the crowded waiting room, with her six year old son on her knee. She is in extreme mental discomfort. After all, how *do* you explain to your doctor that your son shows every sign of developing female breasts? It took a lot of courage for her just to come. What will she do if the doctor laughs at her? She feels embarrassed, and also rather frightened.

But the doctor doesn't laugh. Instead, he asks her, quite seriously, what the boy's been eating. She can't think. She hasn't fed him anything unusual — surely it can't be her fault? Has he been eating veal, the doctor wants to know. His mother thinks . . . yes, he eats veal. It's good white meat, it gives him protein and energy, and he likes the bland taste, because he won't eat other stronger-tasting meat. Why, she asks, what's wrong with it?

The doctor sighs, and tells her. She's not alone. He's seen lots of cases like this recently. Her son is one of over *nine hundred* young boys, aged between six and ten, who show the same symptoms. And there are over *two hundred* young girls — six years of age — who are also affected. That's 1,100 young children, just in Milan, who have begun to develop breasts. The cause? Something about a greedy meat producer, who gave his veal calves too much of a drug called DES . . .

Another place, another connection. This time the setting is Puerto Rico, where in 1979 yet another horrific chapter in the story of DES was about to unfold. The Department of Paediatrics at a local hospital began to find a pattern of disturbing new symptoms amongst its young patients. Like the Milan case, children were starting to show signs of grossly premature sexual development. All the children were under eight years of age, yet they were developing breasts, starting to go through puberty, and show high levels of the human sex hormone oestrogen in their blood. Some of the young girls had ovarian cysts. Some of these symptoms were even seen in girls who were just *six months* old.

Perhaps one of the most poignant symptoms was that many of them had advanced 'bone age'. Growth hormones like DES are known to accelerate the ageing process — and these young people's bodies were getting old before their time. DES was — quite literally — robbing them of their youth.

At first, the authorities tried to deny that DES was the cause of the scandal. The United States Bureau of Veterinary Medicine had despatched a team to Puerto Rico to investigate. They reported that DES just couldn't be the cause of the problem — they'd tried to buy it, but found that it wasn't on sale. In any case, they said, DES had been banned by the authorities since 1979, and consequently it was quite impossible to obtain.

But one local doctor knew differently. She knew that DES was strongly implicated in the disaster, and she set out to prove it. She hired a private detective, and he quickly confirmed that you could buy DES just about everywhere, no questions asked. And it was being used by farmers in a really big way — they thought of it as a 'miracle drug' that boosted their profits no end. It was being used on meat animals, including chickens, right up to the time they were slaughtered. Unfortunately, this is still the case. Horrific cases of childhood abnormalities go on being observed, even today. The nightmare is not yet over for Puerto Rico.

If by now you are feeling angry about this sordid hormone business, you will be even more outraged by the current situation that exists here and now in Great Britain. First, let's reconsider what we've learnt about DES — and remember, this knowledge has been learnt the hard way, by performing experiments on unknowing human subjects.

We know that DES can be a long-term timebomb, whose symptoms may not be revealed for anything up to twenty-nine years after a dose has been received. We know that DES is quite capable of causing cancer and other mutations in the children of women who have been exposed to it during their pregnancy. We also know that DES can cause grossly premature sexual development and ageing in very young children.

So why is it *still* being used by the people who produce our meat?

The Hormone Risk Business

This is the current picture, as it exists in Great Britain and the rest of the European Economic Community, today. DES is not supposed to be used on livestock, although it is common knowledge that it still is. There is even a body of opinion who considers it should *not* be banned. They feel that if DES, and other growth hormones, are totally prohibited — as DES was in Puerto Rico — then a black market will be created, and there will be absolutely no control over the way they are used. They feel that 'controlled use' is best. This would mean not dosing an animal for at least three months before it is slaughtered. It would mean cutting off the animal's ear in the slaughterhouse and destroying it, because this is the place on the animal's body where the injection should be given (although it isn't always). It would also mean that meat producers would have to agree to only use DES and other growth promoters in the doses that are advised. Well, who is naïve enough to believe that all these guidelines will be observed, by all the meat producers, all the time?

But more importantly, *why* should animals be dosed up with growth promoters in any case? There is no clinical or therapeutic reason for doing so. It is certainly not in the interests of the consumer. And it just adds to the already colossal meat mountain within the EEC. But, of course, it is *very much* in the interests of the meat producers. They estimate they can get at least £30 more profit from each cow that has been treated, which means that the British meat industry would lose about £40 million a year if hormones were not used. That's the equivalent of cutting the price of beef by about 4p per pound.

Our bureaucrats, too, are basically opposed to a complete ban on synthetic growth hormones. They say that it would cost about £100 to test just one animal's carcass for DES-type residue. A newly-developed test would bring down the cost to about £5 per carcass, but this is still likely to cost at least £7 million pounds each year — and even that is too much for them. There is also the transatlantic trade to consider. The Americans, who use hormones in a big way, sell over $100 million of beef to European countries every year, and they have threatened 'grave retaliations' if this trade is jeopardized.

Of course, it's not just the meat producers who profit from the use of synthetic growth hormones. The large pharmaceutical companies do as well, although they seem quite confident that there's nothing to worry about. 'If the authorities considered that there was a hazard to the public from misuse,' said one spokesman, 'there would be stricter controls.'[3]

There have been many attempts to get the EEC to impose a total prohibition on the use of growth hormones. Each time, the attempts have been blocked — astonishingly by Great Britain. Mr Michael Jopling, the British Agriculture Secretary, speaking after vetoing yet another proposal, said that the attempts at prohibition were 'Luddite moves in the face of scientific advice.' And Professor Eric Lamming of Nottingham University called the attempted banning 'dangerous and politically motivated,' and felt that a total ban could 'endanger consumers.'[3] He said that farmers would be tempted to obtain hormones anyway, and inject them into meat-bearing parts of animals where they could not be detected. In other words, the consumer has two choices. He or she can either eat meat that is *known* to be 'mildly' contaminated with growth hormones — or he or she can risk eating meat that *may* be *extremely* contaminated with growth hormones. Some choice.

But the situation gets even worse. How many animals are currently dosed with hormones in this country? The answer is that we don't know, because records are not usually kept or collated. One estimate has been made by the Institute for Research in Animal Diseases, who guess that between thirty and fifty per cent of meat intended for domestic consumption has had hormones implanted. Another estimate puts the figure nearer eighty per cent for beef cattle. But no-one can tell for sure.

Surely, you would think, we must be conducting scientific research into the effects of eating meat contaminated with growth hormones on human beings? The answer here is that we *were* doing research, but the government has decided to scrap it. Dr Ray Heitzman, who has been paid by the Ministry of Agriculture to research into the problem, has now had his grant taken away. 'We have been told we are not going to be allowed to work in this area,' said Dr Heitzman. 'I think we are causing more problems than we are solving for some people.'[3]

Winning the Battle But Losing the War

Nevertheless, on the 20 December 1985, the Council of Ministers of the EEC finally agreed to overrule Britain's objection, and gave their approval to a prohibition of the use of growth promoting hormones on meat animals. At last, common sense seemed to have triumphed. The battle had been won, and we could all feel safe again, couldn't we?

Sadly, no. For a start, Britain has obtained special exemption from the ban until 1989. So there's no possibility of any change in this country until then. And then what will happen? It is certain that a massive black market in all types of hormones will still carry on, probably bigger than ever. How do we know this? Because the meat industry themselves say so, quite openly. This is how one of Britain's meat bosses, the Director General of the Meat and Livestock Commission, puts it:

> A blanket ban on the use of a product which people see as being commercially desirable, and which the great majority of people see no problem with, would be certain to drive it underground. That's what happened with alcohol in the United States in the twenties — when it was prohibited everyone traded illicitly and widely, and I suspect the same might happen in this country if there were a total ban on the use of hormones.[4]

There *is* a booming black market in animal growth hormones in this country at this very moment, and it looks as if it's going to get worse. A drug like DES is not difficult to make in an illicit laboratory. The profits make the minimal risk well worthwhile. The basic raw materials come in across the Iron Curtain, usually from Poland, Russia and sometimes China. In April 1985, the Belgian police swooped on an illegal laboratory, and discovered a drug ring employing thirty people, in a business they estimated to be worth £50 million every year. This particular ring was manufacturing DES — and it's certain that at least some of this was intended for the British market.

In most countries, however, there have never been any prosecutions for the illegal manufacture or trading in DES. It seems that the authorities aren't very interested, and in any case there's just not enough manpower on the side of the law to cope. In Britain, the Pharmaceutical Society has a statutory obligation to police the trade in human and animal medicines, but with only a handful of inspectors they face a daunting task. Even so, they have discovered five major drug rings within the last ten years. What happens, you may ask, when a trafficker is caught? In theory, there can be unlimited fines, and up to two years in gaol. But in practice, according to an investigator I spoke to, the usual fine does not exceed a few thousand pounds. And, unlike those who trade in drugs for direct human consumption, no trafficker has ever been sent to gaol.

'It's a tough job to get hard evidence,' one investigator told me. 'No-one likes talking to you, because the farming community sticks together. You get the feeling that no matter how much you manage to uncover, it's still just the tip of the iceberg.'

'What happens to the trafficker when he gets caught?,' I asked.

'One case recently is a good example,' he said. 'The value of the drugs in question was £40,000, but the fine was only £7,500. And there were over 270 T.I.C.s.'

'What's that?,' I asked.

'A T.I.C. means Taken Into Consideration,' he replied. 'It means that the offender asked the court to take over 270 other cases into consideration when sentencing him. So he can't be prosecuted for them now.'

So it seems as if the only group within society who *will* benefit when hormones finally become illegal will be the person who peddles the drugs — and, of course, the meat industry which keeps him in business.

You may have wondered why it is that no tests are performed on the carcasses of animals to establish whether they are contaminated. Well, a few tests are performed. My information is that 300 are carried out every year. Three hundred tests — on an industry that kills and processes *1,400,000 animals each day*. But the Ministry of Agriculture, Fisheries and Food seems quite satisfied with this amount. They say it would be impossible to do any more, because no cheap test has been devised to detect hormones on a larger basis. And it is unlikely that any such test *will* be developed — because the only place of research in the world that *was* developing such a test — the Institute for Research In Animal Diseases — has had its funding cut away.

It's not surprising that the cynics are saying that the European decision to ban hormones has, in reality, more to do with trying to reduce the EEC's massive seventy five thousand tonne beef mountain, than with protecting the legitimate interests of the consumers.

The Darkness Deepens

All these connections are coming together to paint a very dark picture indeed. A chance meeting between two doctors in a hospital lift: the tragic cases of eleven hundred little boys and girls in Milan: a Puerto Rican doctor who was so horrified by what she saw in her surgery that she hired a private detective to investigate: and shabby political manoeuvrings within the EEC.

It is a story of powerful interests acting to protect themselves and their profits, regardless of the true cost to the consumer. In the meat industry, it's a depressingly familiar pattern. By the time you've finished reading this book, it's quite likely that many of your preconceptions about meat (and about the people who sell it) will have been shattered. We tend to think of it as a 'pure' food, possessing a high degree of nourishment, and virtually an indispensible part of the modern diet. So, of course, when we learn about it being contaminated with a substance such as DES, we are quite naturally shocked.

In fact, though, this image of meat as being 'essential' and 'wholesome' is a relatively recent one, owing much to the long periods of scarcity when meat was virtually unobtainable both during and after the second world war — a period which, ironically, was one of the healthiest in recent British history. So let's continue by taking a close look at this 'mythology' of meat, and find out just how close it is to reality . . .

REFERENCES

1. *The Lancet*, 2/9/78 'Dangers of Diethyl Stilboestrol', p. 520, Brackbill and Berendes.
2. *Clinical Oncology*, 1977,3,75-80, 'Stilboestrol and Human Cancer', Bishun, Smith and Williams.
3. *The Guardian*, 15/11/85, 20/11/85, 19/11/85.
4. 'Good Enough To Eat?', Thames Television 1985.

Also see:

The Lancet, 27/3/82, 'Anabolics in Meat Production', p. 721.
British Journal of Obstetrics and Gynaecology, March 1981, Vol 88, pp 322-326, 'A case of clear cell adenocarcinoma of the vagina in pregnancy', Davis, Wadehra, McIntosh, Monaghan.
The New England Journal of Medicine, February 13th 1975, 292:334-339, 'Prenatal Exposure to Stilboestrol', Herbst, Poskanzer, Robboy, Friendlander, Scully.
The Lancet, 17/1/76, p. 152, 'Prenatal Diethyl Stilboestrol exposure and male hypogonadism', Hoefnagel.
The New Statesman, 'Swallow it Whole', Wright, 16/7/82.
The Economist, 'Down on the Pharm', 27/3/82.

*For the latest development see item on page 232 about hormone growth promoters.

2

Meat-eaters or Wheat-eaters

Most people probably have a question something like this buried deep inside their subconscious mind —

'Isn't it the natural thing for us to do to eat meat?'

The answer to this is, quite simply, 'No'. There is nothing at all natural about the quantity or quality of meat that is included in the average Western diet these days. Even so, most people have the image in their minds that humans are somehow genetically programmed to eat flesh foods, and cannot thrive without them. So what about our ancestors? How did *they* live?

They probably originated in the East African Rift Valley, which is a dry and desolate place today, but would have been very different two to four million years ago. The habitat was very lush then. There were large, shallow freshwater lakes, with rich open grassland on the flood plains and dense woodland beside the rivers. Fossil evidence shows that foodstuffs such as Leguminosae (peas and beans) and Anacardiacae (cashew nuts) were readily available, as were Palmae (sago, dates, and coconuts). Evidence gained from the analysis of tooth markings indicates that our ancestors' diet was much the same as the Guinea Baboon's is today — hard seeds, stems, some roots, plant fibre — a typically tough diet requiring stripping, chopping and chewing actions.

Our ancestors also had very large molars, with small incisors, unsuited to meat consumption but ideal for consuming large quantities of vegetable matter. By 2.5 million years B.C., however, evidence shows that the land began to dry out, forcing Australopithecus (the name of our early ancestor) to desert this idyllic 'Garden of Eden' and try and survive on the savannas, where they were poorly prepared for the evolutionary struggle that was to come.

Before this crucial point, there is no doubt that our ancestors had largely followed a meatless diet typical of primates, with a few eggs and insects thrown in occasionally. The zoologist Desmond Morris made an interesting observation about this period in our development, in his book *The Naked Ape*, when he wrote:

> It could be argued that, since our primate ancestors had to make do without a major meat component in their diets, we should be able to do the same. We were driven to become flesh eaters only by environmental circumstances, and now that we have the environment under control, with elaborately cultivated crops at our disposal, we might be expected to return to our ancient primate feeding patterns. [1]

So we became omnivorous — we were *forced* by our rapidly changing environment to eat anything and everything we could get our hands on. Which included some flesh foods. So to what degree did we consume meat?

Omnivores — Not Carnivores

As our old habitat receded, we had to make some quick decisions. We had been used to eating a mainly fruit and nut diet. As this became increasingly scarce, we had to adapt to eating whatever we could find. There wasn't much. We found roots and grasses, and made do with them. We would have stumbled across some partly-rotten carrion flesh, and gratefully eaten what we could salvage. We would have chased easy-to-catch small game. We ate it all, no questions asked. Interestingly, we still preserve some ability to digest and utilize leaves and grasses, which recent scientific work has discovered, and probably dates from this period of our existence. We became not carnivores, but omnivores. We became a jack of all trades, and, this new workload forced our brains to grow and grow. By now, we were no longer typical primates, but we were certainly not typical carnivores either, as this comparison shows:

TYPICAL PRIMATE	TYPICAL CARNIVORE	OMNIVORE HUMANS
Exists largely on a fruit and nut diet	Consumes flesh exclusively	Able to exist on a mixed diet depending on environment, highly adaptable
Large brains able to exhibit elementary rationalization	Small brains less capable of adaptive behaviour	Large brains, highly adaptable capable of abstract rationalization
Grasping hands capable of using weapons	No manual dexterity	Highly dextrous
Understands role of tools and how to make them	Does not use tools	Sophisticated tool makers/ users
Rudimentary degree of co-operation	Advanced co-operation and hunting in packs	Highly organized and co-operative
Inoffensive excrement, few special rituals	Putrid excrement defecation localized	Offensive excrement many rituals
Continuous feeders living hand to mouth	Large meals infrequently taken	Combines both snack feeding and large meals
Wandering lifestyle, go where the food is	Fixed homebase, food brought back to share with family	Highly territorial
Predominantly sweet-toothed	Predominantly salty/fatty preference	Likes both sweet items and salty and fatty food
Likes to savour food, experiment with variety, combine flavours	Eats food quickly sticks to one taste will not experiment with flavours	Aims not to bolt food down, will tend to experiment

Adaptability is the Key to Our Success

You can see from the table that it is therefore completely wrong to describe our parentage as 'carnivorous'. Some of our characteristics are partly carnivorous, but also, many of them are quite definitely primate, and therefore non-meat eating. The truth lies somewhere between these two extremes — we have become supremely *adaptable*, and have learnt how to survive in almost any environment, no matter how seemingly hostile. In fact, if we as a species can be characterised by just one word, it would be 'adaptability'. It is our passport for success in any situation, no matter how desperate, and unquestionably the key to our survival. We were forced out of our original habitat, and miraculously we survived. We were forced to learn how to live on the plains in fierce competition with natural carnivores, and again we met the challenge.

There are still societies in existence today who lead very similar lives to those of our ancestors, and it is useful to study their way of life, because it gives many clues about our own past. The Bush People of the Kalahari live in just such a society, which has hardly changed in structure for many thousands of years (although it is changing pretty fast today, as they disappear into the so-called 'tribal homelands' of Southern Africa). Apart from modern interference, their society has been so durable precisely because it worked very well. Recently, their lifestyle was subject to an intensive two year study.[2]

For part of the time, there was a serious drought — a life-threatening situation, causing what the sociologists term 'stress'. Surrounding tribes who had (by our definition) 'progressed' to a system of fixed agriculture were almost totally devastated, but the Bush People's lifestyle allowed them to adapt and they were virtually unaffected. Meat, being rarer and more 'costly' to them than plant food, was highly prized and often the centre of their male rituals.

Despite this, by far their most important source of food came from vegetables. Out of eleven males in the encampment, four never went hunting. The other seven males would spend a total of seventy-eight man-days hunting, managing to kill eighteen animals. Their chance of obtaining meat on any one day was about one in four, or twenty-five per cent. By contrast, the women *always* returned from their gathering expeditions with food — a 100 per cent success rate. The entire tribe could comfortably feed itself if each member put in a fifteen hour week — rather better than our own society's achievement.

Meat is a Scarce, Luxury Food

It is quite obvious that, in societies such as these, meat was something of a rare luxury. It would take an area of about forty square miles to provide enough wild game to keep a group of four people fed, and, with such a large territory to cover, there must have been many times when the men returned home without any food.

The importance of vegetable sources of food is confirmed by an analysis of calorie yields (energy) of food obtained. For every hour a woman spent gathering food, she produced two and a half times as many food calories as every hour a man spent hunting.

To characterize societies such as these as 'hunting' societies seems to be extremely unfair on the women — who provide the majority of the (vegetable) food, and it gives the hunting males rather more credit for being 'providers' than they should fairly have. Perhaps in our assessment of such societies, we have been more impressed with the rituals and paraphernalia of the male hunter than with the uncomplaining and unrecognized hard work of the females which, quite clearly, is the key to survival of the whole society. It seems likely that the real heroes of our Stone Age period were the women, not the men.

So our ancestors ate much more plant food than is popularly believed. But when agriculture developed, the amount of vegetable food in the diet increased even more — comprising anything up to *ninety per cent* of their total intake of food. This is one big difference between our modern diet and our 'original' diet.

Paradoxically, some people today feel worried that their bodies are somehow biologically 'programmed' to eat meat, and if they don't get it, they'll be unhealthy. In fact, the exact opposite is closer to the truth. We can scientifically prove that human genes have changed very, very little for several tens of thousands of years. But, of course, our diet *has* changed — unfortunately, for the worse.

Basically, our bodies are still in the Stone Age, and expect the sort of nutrition they were getting then. They're just not used to getting the kind of junk food we give them today. No wonder so many diseases are related to our modern pattern of food consumption.

Today's Meat is Nothing Like Primitive Meat

Another big difference between our ancestors' diet and the food we eat today is not just in the *quantity* of meat consumed, but also its *quality*.[3] Modern food animals are bred to be fat: the carcass of a slaughtered animal can easily be thirty per cent fat or more. But the sort of animal that primitive people hunted was a wild animal — it had, on average, only 3.9 per cent fat on its carcass. So today, even if we cut our meat consumption back to the greatly reduced amount that our ancestors consumed, we will still be taking in *seven times* more fat!

But even this isn't the end of the story. The *type* of fat on the carcass of the animal that our ancestors ate was different, as well. Primitive meat had *five times more* polyunsaturated fat in it than today's meat does, which is high in saturated fat, but much lower in polyunsaturated. You can begin to see how very different the two diets are.

And here are some other important differences. Our ancestral diet only had one sixth the amount of sodium (salt) that the modern diet contains. Because fresh food comprised such an important part of the diet, the primitive diet was much, much richer in natural vitamins. For example — there would have been nearly *nine* times as much Vitamin C in the primitive diet. And twice as much fibre. And three times as much total polyunsaturated fat. And so on . . .

So if you were worried that a meat-free diet might not be healthy, don't be. In point of fact, it's much closer to the kind of natural food that we've always eaten, and that our bodies have *always* been used to. The fact is that in terms of quantity and quality, today's meat is nothing like the primitive food that our ancestors would occasionally eat. In evolutionary terms, the meat we eat today is a *new* food for us. This means that we're actually conducting a huge experiment on our own bodies. And so far, the results don't look good . . .

REFERENCES

1.   *The Naked Ape*, Morris, Jonathan Cape, 1967.
2.   'Medical Research Amongst the !Kung', Truswell and Hanson, in *Kalahari Hunter-gatherers*, ed. Lee, DeVore, Harvard University Press, 1976.
3.   'Paleolithic Nutrition: A consideration of its nature and current implications', Eaton, Konner, *New England Journal of Medicine*, Vol 312 No 5, pp. 283-289.

3

Meat, You and Cancer

In evolutionary terms, our bodies are not used to the massive quantities of meat that we've been feeding them. Neither are they used to the large levels of fat, protein and other ingredients that are a necessary part of today's meat-orientated diet. So it's not altogether surprising if, sometimes, things go wrong.

In this chapter, I'm going to present you with the most up-to-date evidence that suggests that meat is causatively-related to certain forms of human cancers. I make no apology for the length of the evidence — the subject is a serious one and has not generally been given enough exposure. I've used a number of specially-constructed computer charts and graphs because they'll help you to quickly understand the main conclusions. If, however, you don't want to read all the evidence, simply skip to the verdict at the end of the chapter, where the main evidence is summarized.

The Risk

Although the word 'cancer' is no longer an automatic death sentence, it still has the power to fill most of us with an unspeakable dread. For cancer is probably the most feared of all diseases. And it is virtually inevitable that we will have close personal contact with it at sometime in our lives — perhaps through a friend, a close relative, or even first-hand experience.

Cancer and the human race are old enemies. Various civilizations have suffered from it since at least Egyptian days (traces of the disease have been found in mummies taken from the pyramids).

Despite our long acquaintance with it, it is still regarded as a malevolent and mysterious illness by many people. And indeed, we are right to be deeply concerned by it. Because, although we are getting better and better at *treating* the disease, we've made virtually no progress towards *preventing* it. In the United Kingdom there has been a stubborn rise in deaths attributable to cancer over the last 35 years:[1]

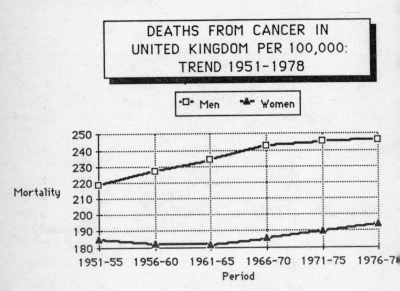

Warning Signs

Growing public awareness of the epidemic nature of the problem has undoubtedly resulted in earlier diagnosis and treatment, which, despite everything, is still our main weapon against the disease. The importance of early treatment cannot be overemphasized. The American Cancer Society suggests there are seven warning signs which, even if only one is present, should prompt a quick investigation. They are:

- Unusual bleeding or discharge
- Appearance of a lump or swelling
- Hoarseness of cough
- Indigestion or difficulty in swallowing
- Change in bowel or bladder habits
- A sore that does not heal
- A change in a wart or mole

Cancer as a Cause of Death

While the incidence of cancers (sometimes referred to as 'neoplasms') in the West has been increasing over recent years, certain other causes of mortality, such as infectious diseases, have been successfully fought. This means that cancer-related deaths figure much more prominently now than they ever have previously as a cause of death. Indeed, in many Western countries cancer is now the number one cause of mortality. This chart illustrates the situation in the United States, which is fairly typical:

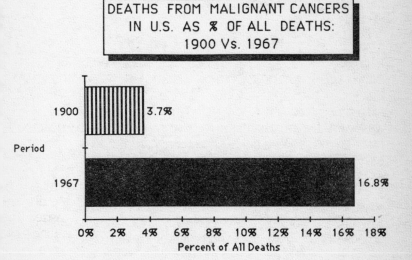

DEATHS FROM MALIGNANT CANCERS
IN U.S. AS % OF ALL DEATHS:
1900 Vs. 1967

1900 3.7%

Period

1967 16.8%

0% 2% 4% 6% 8% 10% 12% 14% 16% 18%
Percent of All Deaths

What Do We Mean by 'Cancer'?

There are more than 150 types of cancer, each exhibiting different characteristics. The essential feature is a disorganized growth of cells, that may occur anywhere in the body, which multiply and may eventually destroy their host. Malignant forms will invade other cells, and use the body's circulatory system to migrate to any part of the body (a process called metastasis). Benign forms do not exhibit this aggressive 'behaviour'. Because of this ability to invade and destroy healthy parts of the body, the Greek doctor Hippocrates called it '*karkinos*', literally meaning 'a crab', from which the modern word cancer is derived.

Cancers are broadly divided into two main types — carcinomas and sarcomas. A carcinoma is a disease affecting the tissues that cover both the external and internal body, for example, breast cancer, prostate cancer, or cancer of the uterus. A sarcoma, on the other hand, is a disease that affects the body's connective tissue, such as muscles, blood vessels, and bone. The prospects for survival depend, amongst other things, on the site in the body affected, the speed of diagnosis, the treatment given, and perhaps even on the attitude of the patient towards the disease.

What Causes Cancer?

It has been recently estimated that up to sixty per cent of all cancers in the Western world today may be related to environmental factors.[2] But, in fact, this isn't a new idea. As long ago as 1775 the eminent surgeon Sir Percivall Pott suggested that there might be a link. Pott was one of the great names in the history of medicine. He was the first to notice how chimney sweeps often developed a particular form of cancer, and put forward the theory that their atrocious working conditions were responsible.

So if we have reason to suspect that our environment *might* be a factor in the causation of cancer, shouldn't we try to do something to control it, or at least to reduce the risk? After all, we spend huge amounts of money trying to find cures or ore effective treatments for cancer. Surely we should also be trying to *prevent* the disease from appearing in the first place?

Unfortunately, this path is not so easy. In theory, we should be able to isolate and control risk factors in our environment. But in practice, there are many artificially-created problems to overcome. Such as persistent and highly successful lobbying from tobacco manufacturers, for example, which is undoubtedly the major cause of lung cancer (the most common form, accounting for twenty-seven per cent of all cancer-related deaths in males, and twenty-two per cent in females). Another problem is the lack of sufficient public funds to ensure widespread public health education and awareness. One day the sad truth will finally emerge — that our politicians, who have the immense power to alter a nation's health for the better, were too self-interested to bother. We will have been badly served.

Cancer in Our Diet?

In 1981 an epoch-making report was produced by the eminent epidemiologists Richard Doll and Richard Peto.[3] It assembled all the evidence they could find linking the occurrence of human cancers to specific identifiable factors. While the authors of the 1308-page report warn that not all causes of cancer can either be identified or avoided, it does seem from the evidence they collected that *some* of the causes of cancer they identify *are well within our own control*. This is what they estimate the main risk factors to be, with their best estimate of the percentage of total cancer-caused deaths that are attributable to them:

FACTOR RESPONSIBLE FOR CANCER	PERCENTAGE OF ALL DEATHS
Diet	35
Tobacco	30
Infection	10
Reproductive and Sexual Behaviour	7
Occupation	4
Alcohol	3

FACTOR RESPONSIBLE FOR CANCER	PERCENTAGE OF ALL DEATHS
Geophysical Factors	3
Pollution	2
Food Additives	1
Industrial Products	1
Medicines and Medical Products	1

You can see that 'Diet' comes right at the top of the list. 'Diet' means what we *choose* to eat, doesn't it? So, by informing ourselves of the evidence, and by taking steps to change our diets accordingly, we *ought* to be able to significantly reduce our chances of suffering from a diet-related cancer, oughtn't we? There's just one problem, of course. The food industry doesn't necessarily want us to change.

The Food Industry Opposes the Public Interest

While our politicians may be complacent to the point of negligence, the real villains of the piece are the people within the food industry who actually act, on occasion, against the public interest. Quite simply, they do not want their customers to change their food habits and will fight very hard indeed to hold on to their market. You can see a good example of this in Britain's dairy industry. A recent government report[4] at last suggested that the British people should, for their own health, reduce the amount of animal fat in their diet, from the present very high level of 40 per cent of all calories by a mere 5 per cent to 35 per cent of calories. A mild enough proposal, when you learn that the World Health Organisation advises that no more than 10 per cent of dietary calories should come from saturated animal fat. But even this small change — of only 5 per cent — would mean that Britain's dairy herd would have to be reduced to one half of its present size.

You can see why the food industry (in this case, the powerful dairy industry) doesn't really want things to change. Their solution is much more profit-orientated — they want us to drink even *more* milk, not less!

'Liquid milk consumption on the domestic market could be increased above current levels', says the Milk Marketing Board's general manager for marketing. 'It is not just a question of telling the housewife to order an extra pinta on the doorstep. You should go into your local pub and ask the landlord to put on milk for sale. Equally three and a half million cans of Coke are drunk every day in this country. I wouldn't mind fifty per cent of that market with flavoured milk drinks.'[5]

And the meat trade is just the same. Take pork pies, for instance, which are a massive source of saturated fat. This is what a director of one of Britain's biggest supermarket chains thinks about pork pies:

'The bad news', he said recently when addressing a meat industry conference, 'is that a pork pie is a ball of meat with a fairly high fat content, wrapped in an envelope of fatty pastry.'

So are we going to see pork pies disappear from his supermarket's shelves, and replaced with healthier food in the public interest? No, not at all. This is how he continued:

'The good news is that people enjoy pork pies and will continue to do so. Logic might anticipate the demise of the pork pie, but *we* must not. We only need to keep half a step ahead of our customers. Keeping a whole step ahead is called a self-fulfilling prophecy and has no place in intelligent marketing.'[6]

The Meat Industry Fights Dirty

There are many ways that the meat industry can successfully oppose any change in consumers' buying habits, and you should know about them so that you can recognize them. The first of many weapons available to them is their ability to create a confusing smokescreen in the public's mind. The keyword here is the word 'debate'. Call it the fat 'debate', or the meat 'debate'. Immediately, it implies that the subject is confusing, that there are many different viewpoints, and no-one really knows the truth. And it makes it very difficult for consumers to know who to believe. So they do nothing — which is precisely what the industry wants.

It also has the effect of relegating scientific evidence to the level of personal opinion. Objective facts become personal viewpoints, which, of course, carry much less weight. It becomes a tit-for-tat battle, with no winners, and only one loser — the public. The overall aim is to create so much *confusion* in the public's mind that they are unsure, indecisive, and ultimately do not change their food habits. It is a very successful technique.

Another tactic they are using with increasing frequency is to abuse and belittle their opponents. This is not always so effective. After a time, the public may begin to wonder why they are acting so defensively. What have they got to hide? In just the past year or so, the meat industry has called its opponents 'extreme groups,' and has accused them of spreading 'extremist propaganda,' (in the words of the head of Britain's Meat and Livestock Commission). [7] The meat industry has also accused its opponents of 'circulating inaccurate information and distortion' (in other words, lying). Its opponents have been called 'inaccurate, racialist and offensive,' by the managing director of one of Britain's largest chain of butchers. [8] The meat industry also tries to scare the public about the 'pitfalls of extremism and cranky diets.' The Meat and Livestock Commission calls its opponents 'groups with extreme opinions, representing a tiny minority of the population, who make a great deal of noise, and fire a barrage of unbalanced propaganda.' [9]

So, although there is still much scientific work yet to do on the ultimate causes of human cancer, don't be misled by the meat industry into thinking that the whole area is shrouded in darkness and confusion. *We know much more than they would have you believe.* So let's recognize the tactics of the meat industry for what they are, and take a long, hard look at this product that they are so desperately trying to keep us eating . . .

Meat — the First Clue

As researchers studied facts and figures about mortality from cancer in different countries, they were struck by an odd fact. It seemed that certain countries had a much higher mortality rate than others. What was the factor that made the United States, for example, so much worse than Japan? The researchers looked for a clue. Then, they tried comparing the amount of animal protein that different nations ate with their cancer mortality.[10] This is what they began to see:

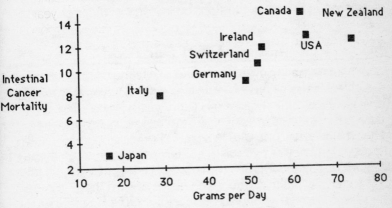

ANIMAL PROTEIN INTAKE COMPARED TO CANCER MORTALITY

There certainly seemed to be a clear relationship between the amount of animal protein in the national diet and the incidence of certain forms of cancer mortality. But this wasn't the only connection. The same 'straight-line' connection seemed to exist between *total* fat consumption and cancer, *animal* fat consumption and cancer, and various other linked factors as well. This was surely compelling evidence, wasn't it?

Well it was strongly suggestive, but it wasn't necessarily conclusive. For one thing, scientists are taught to be extremely cautious. Before coming to any firm conclusion they must painstakingly check their data, be alert to errors, biases, and unrepresentative samples. Then they have to be able to duplicate their findings, not just once, but again and again. And then, of course, they have to attempt to understand what their findings actually mean, and test various hypotheses that might explain them.

All this takes a long time. Take the issue of cigarette tobacco, for example. Most of us have known that smoking is the major cause of lung cancer, and other severe diseases, for a long time. But to actually *prove* it scientifically has taken over twenty-five years. And even now, cigarette manufacturers still do not accept that smoking causes lung cancer. As the case went before the American courts, in an attempt to sue one tobacco manufacturer for making a defective product, the lead attorney for the tobacco company (R. J. Reynolds) would not concede that smoking causes cancer. 'It is an open scientific question,' he says.[11]

Cancer From Our Food?

Despite mounting evidence,[12] it was still just possible, of course, that diet had nothing to do with it. There might have been another hidden factor, which everyone up till then had overlooked. Perhaps certain nations were genetically more likely to contract cancers, no matter what they ate?

To examine this possibility, studies were undertaken amongst immigrant populations. If the cause of cancer was genetic rather than environmental, the same races should have the same occurrence of cancers, wherever they lived. The Japanese seemed to be a good subject, because they traditionally had low incidence of most forms of cancer (with a few exceptions, such as stomach cancer). So three groups of Japanese were chosen, together with a 'control' group of Caucasians.

The first group of Japanese lived in Japan, and followed a largely traditional diet. The second group lived in the United States, but had been born abroad. The third group lived in the States and had been born there. The graph opposite shows what they found.[13]

The results speak for themselves. A comparison between the extreme left and right columns shows that the Japanese living in Japan (left column) have only one quarter the risk of contracting cancer of the colon as Caucasian Americans living in the States. But even more significantly, when the Japanese *move* to the States, their chance of contracting cancer of the colon increases by three times — almost the same risk as a Caucasian. The place of birth didn't seem to matter. This was good proof that environmental, and not genetic, factors were indeed very significant.

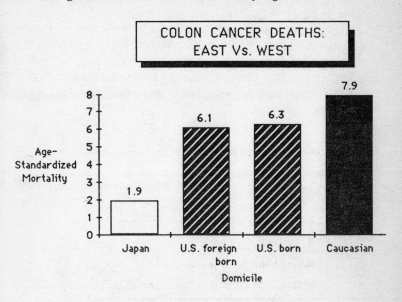

The focus began to shift from international comparisons, which had pointed the way, to very specific studies amongst closely similar groups. Similar, that is, except for one or two key factors, which could be isolated, studied, and perhaps even controlled.

Cancer from Which Part of Our Diet?

And now the scientific detective work really began. Because if the environment — probably diet — really was so important, then it should be possible to track down which specific factors related most strongly to increasing cancer risk, and, hopefully, try to control them.

The focus began to shift from international comparisons, which had pointed the way, to very specific studies amongst closely similar groups. Similar, that is, except for one or two key factors, which could be isolated, studied, and perhaps even controlled.

A group that was quickly identified as being of particular interest was the American Seventh Day Adventist population. This group was subject to repeated studies, because the feature that distinguished them from the general American population was their differing diet. One key area of difference is dramatically demonstrated in this chart:[14]

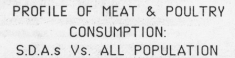

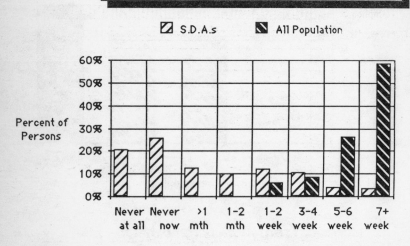

The Chart shows that Seventh Day Adventists eat a completely different diet to the average American one. The vast majority of the general population use meat or poultry products seven or more times each week, but the picture is quite the reverse for the Seventh Day Adventist group. About half of them *don't* consume meat or meat products. They do not smoke or drink (although in the survey one-third of the men were previous smokers) and they tend to practise a 'healthy' lifestyle that emphasises fresh fruits, whole grains, vegetables and nuts. Certainly a different way of eating compared to the majority of people.

So now the scientists had found a good group of people to study. A major seven year scientific survey, lasting from 1958 to 1965.[15]

followed a large group of 35,460 Adventists and tabulated their cause of death. This is part of their findings:

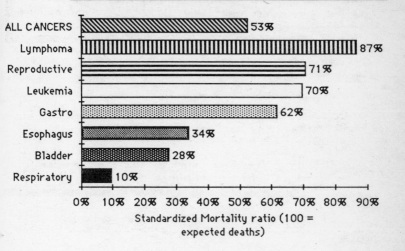

DEATHS FROM CANCER IN S.D.As COMPARED TO GENERAL POPULATION

ALL CANCERS — 53%
Lymphoma — 87%
Reproductive — 71%
Leukemia — 70%
Gastro — 62%
Esophagus — 34%
Bladder — 28%
Respiratory — 10%

Standardized Mortality ratio (100 = expected deaths)

Some Astonishing Results

They found that the death-rate from *all* cancers among Adventists was amazingly almost *half* that of the general population. The top bar on the chart shows this — Adventists only having fifty-three per cent as many deaths from cancer when compared to the norm. Some of this could probably be attributed to their abstinence from smoking — cancer of the respiratory system, for example (the bottom bar on the chart), only being 10 per cent of the general population's. But other cancers, such as gastrointestinal and reproductive ones, are not causatively related to smoking. One of the studies stated:

'It is quite clear that these results are supportive of the hypothesis that beef, meat, and saturated fat or fat in general are etiologically related to colon cancer.'[14]

More Nails in Meat's Coffin

Another study set out to confirm these amazing findings, and ran from 1960 through to 1972.[16] In this one, cancers of the large bowel, breast and prostate were studied — the three most common ones that are *unrelated* to smoking.

Twenty thousand Seventh Day Adventists were studied, and this time, they were compared to two other population groups. Firstly, they were checked against cancer mortality figures for *all* U.S. whites, and then they were compared to a special group of 113,000 people who were chosen because their lifestyle closely matched the Adventists — except, that is, for their diet. In other respects, such as place of residence, income and socio-economic status, the third group was very closely matched to the Adventists. This is how the picture looked:

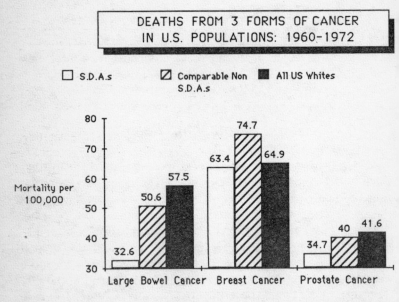

DEATHS FROM 3 FORMS OF CANCER
IN U.S. POPULATIONS: 1960–1972

☐ S.D.A.s   ▨ Comparable Non   ■ All US Whites
                         S.D.A.s

Mortality per 100,000

	Large Bowel Cancer	Breast Cancer	Prostate Cancer
S.D.A.s	32.6	63.4	34.7
Comparable Non S.D.A.s	50.6	74.7	40
All US Whites	57.5	64.9	41.6

Once again, the results looked pretty dramatic. The Adventists are shown on the chart by the white column, and the general population by the black column. The shaded column represents the special group whose lifestyle closely matched the Adventists — apart from the food they ate. You can see that for all three cancers, deaths among the Adventists were *much* lower than for the other groups. It is interesting that there does not appear to be a very great reduction in the risk of breast cancer among Adventists — until, that is, you compare the Adventists results with those of the comparable group (shaded in the chart). The comparable group has a *higher* risk of contracting breast cancer than the national average (probably due to local environmental factors in California, where the study was undertaken). However, the Adventists have succeeded in reducing their own risk back down to below the national average — even though only half of them *never* consume meat.

Zen and the Art of Avoiding Cancer

Yet another study — this time among Zen Buddhist priests — continued to confirm the emerging pattern. The study[17] was undertaken over twenty-four years, and compared mortality amongst Zen priests to the population as a whole. Traditionally, Zen monks abstained from drinking, smoking and meat-eating on religious principles.

These days, however, they are allowed to marry, and can eat meat, drink and smoke, although in fact they do so much less than the general population, which makes them worth studying. In fact, less than ten per cent of the priests actually ate meat on a daily basis, whereas fifty per cent of the general Japanese population eat it every day.

However, seventy per cent of the Zen priests ate fresh vegetables every day. By now, it should come as no surprise to you to learn that, over a broad spread of diseases, the Zen priests looked in much better shape. Compared to the general population, they had significantly less mortality from diabetes, from all forms of cerebrovascular causes, from heart diseases, from ulcers, and from all forms of cancer. Once again, it provided good evidence that your diet *can* affect your health, and particularly your susceptibility to certain common types of cancer.

A Major Study Shows the Risk Foods

We're starting to build a general picture of the relationship between animal flesh in the diet and certain forms of cancers. But we still need to know what the main risk factors are. Wouldn't it be a good idea to try and *isolate* specific dietary factors? This is precisely what many scientists thought, too.

In order to do this, it is necessary to see whether there is a connection between specific components of a diet, such as meat fat, calories from meat, etc., and deaths from a particular type of cancer. This connection is worked out statistically, and is called a correlation.

It's really quite simple. A correlation ends up as a number somewhere in-between minus one and plus one — never more or less than those two figures. The *higher* the figure, the closer the connection between the two factors. For example, if someone is paid on a hourly basis, then the more they work, the more money they earn. This is an example of a *perfect* correlation, and would have a figure of +1.

On the other hand, the more money you spend, the less you have in your bank account — this is a perfect *negative* correlation, since the connection between greater spending and a low bank balance is an inverse one: in this case, the correlation would be −1. And if any two factors, such as today's temperature and your bank balance, are not related at all, then the correlation would have a figure of zero. So the closer the figure gets to *either* +1 or −1, the stronger the connection.

A major correlation study analysed the diets of thirty-seven nations between 1964 and 1966, and then correlated the components of the diets to mortality from cancer of the intestines.[18] The next chart has been drawn from the information it revealed.

You can see that *all* the meat factors correlate very strongly with cancer of the intestines. Total calories, total protein, and total fat

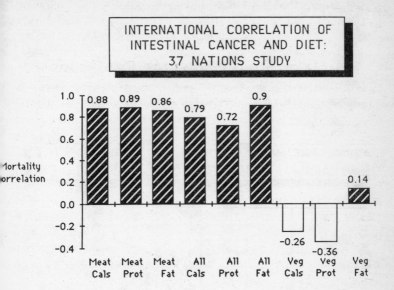

INTERNATIONAL CORRELATION OF
INTESTINAL CANCER AND DIET:
37 NATIONS STUDY

Mortality correlation

Also correlate strongly, which is not surprising, since meat is heavy in all three. But calories and protein from vegetable sources have a *negative* correlation — in other words, they appear to give some form of protection. The study concluded: 'Animal sources of food were clearly associated with the cancer rates.'

Correlation studies like this are very important, because although we may not know precisely *why* and *how* meat in the diet contributes to various cancers (this may take many years to finally prove), we can at least see that there is a clear relationship — and this enables those of us who want to take the necessary precautions for our own wellbeing.

Cancer Doubles in Israel as Meat-Eating Soars

More data, this time from an Israeli study,[19] revealed a connection between both fats from animal sources and fats from plant sources, suggesting that saturated and even unsaturated fats may be connected with increased mortality. The study followed the Jewish population as it grew from 1.17 million in 1949 to 3.5 million in 1975, over which period fat consumption shot up by fifty-two per cent, meat consumption increased by 454 per cent, and the death rate from malignant cancers doubled. You can see how deaths from cancers rose in proportion to the amount of animal fat in the diet.

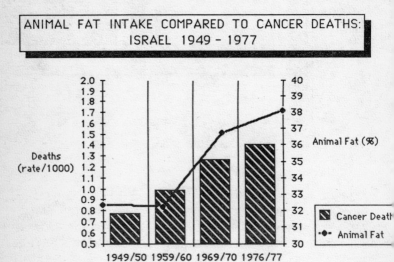

ANIMAL FAT INTAKE COMPARED TO CANCER DEATHS: ISRAEL 1949 - 1977

As the amount of animal fat in the diet shot up, so did the number of people dying from cancer. The same study produced another correlation between specific foods and mortality due to all forms of cancer. They found that cereals, fish and potatoes seemed to give some protection, but sugar, eggs, oils and — worst of all — meat were all associated with increased deaths from cancer. This is how it looks graphically:

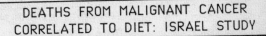

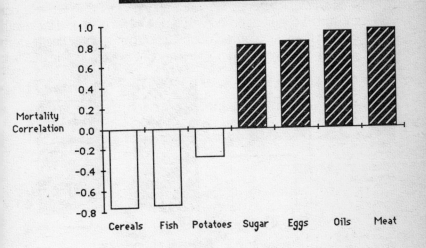

DEATHS FROM MALIGNANT CANCER
CORRELATED TO DIET: ISRAEL STUDY

Meat and Breast Cancer

More and more evidence was starting to accumulate. In Alberta, Canada, researchers compared the diets of women with breast cancer to a control group without the disease.[20] This study was on the look out for a correlation between breast cancer and specific foods, in particular, animal-derived ones. After analysing the data, they were able to show that the risk of contracting breast cancer increases with the amount of beef and pork in the diet:

For pork, an intake of anything more than once a week is associated with a *doubling* of the risk of contracting this form of cancer. The study concluded: 'The results suggest an association between breast cancer and the consumption of beef and pork. These findings are consistent with the higher breast cancer rates in areas of the world with higher per capita beef and pork availability'.

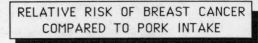

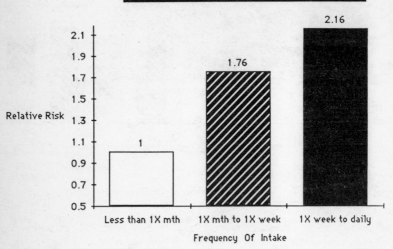

RELATIVE RISK OF BREAST CANCER COMPARED TO PORK INTAKE

Frequency Of Intake

In Hawaii another study showed the same pattern.[21] The study concentrated on a representative sample of the whole of Hawaii's residents — Caucasians, Japanese, Chinese, Filipinos, and, of course, Hawaiians. The wide variety of ethnic groups was useful, since it included a particularly wide range of food habits. Significant associations were established between:

- Breast cancer and all forms of fat and animal protein.
- Cancer of the uterus and all forms of fat and animal protein.
- Prostate cancer and fat and animal protein.

The positive correlations between various forms of food and breast cancer are shown in the next chart, and the only *negative* correlation is between breast cancer and complex carbohydrates — which are found in plants, indicating that plant food may have some form of protective effect:

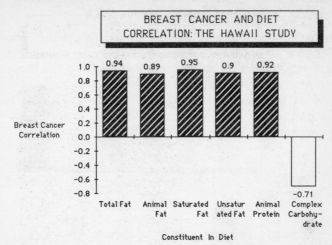

Once more, a very high correlation with all forms of fat and animal protein — and meat is, of course, primarily animal fat and animal protein. But also, another significantly *negative* correlation with complex carbohydrates, such as plant foods. And almost exactly the same relationship emerged when the same study examined cancer of the uterus:

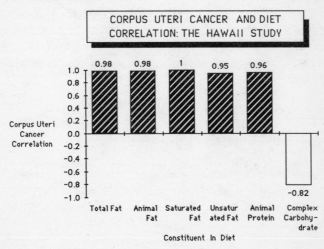

Meat Means More Risk

In 1981 yet another massive statistical world survey of 41 countries (including the U.S. and the U.K.) was completed.[22] The results confirm the connection between eating meat, and risk of certain types of cancer. And yet again, they also show that plant foods seem to confer some protection. These are two charts drawn from data that the survey produced:

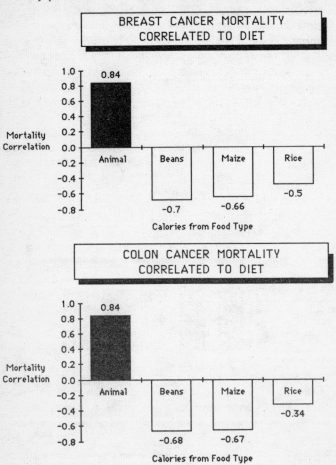

BREAST CANCER MORTALITY
CORRELATED TO DIET

Mortality Correlation

Animal 0.84
Beans −0.7
Maize −0.66
Rice −0.5

Calories from Food Type

COLON CANCER MORTALITY
CORRELATED TO DIET

Mortality Correlation

Animal 0.84
Beans −0.68
Maize −0.67
Rice −0.34

Calories from Food Type

Breast cancer is, of course, the most common form of female cancer, and cancer of the colon is a very common cancer amongst men. A survey of such a size cannot take account of regional fluctuations, but that isn't so important. What is important is that it reveals a very broad, international trend, which many millions of people have in common. The authors of the survey speculate that the *negative* correlation between plant foods such as beans and maize and these forms of cancer may indicate that they help in some way to protect against cancer. Of course, it is also possible that just the absence of meat from the diet is sufficient to produce this effect. 'It is a question', the report says, 'that may never be resolved, but its resolution becomes somewhat academic when one thinks that in the past dietary changes in human populations simultaneously have reduced starchy foods and increased meat consumption. This may indicate that disease prevention could be accomplished by reversing both trends simultaneously. The role of starchy vegetables may be to satisfy the appetite and, therefore, limit the excessive meat intake.'

The report draws a number of straightforward conclusions. It says that total fat and animal protein (i.e., meat) 'strongly correlate internationally with arteriosclerotic heart disease, colon cancer and breast cancer.'

Referring to Western-style diets, it also says that: 'Meat consumption appears to be excessive when compared to other countries and when compared to nutritional requirements'.

Finally, it recommends that meat consumption should be reduced in order to reverse the trends of high cancer rates. It sounds like good advice.

Change Your Diet — Save Your Life

So what actually happens when you start to change your diet? A clue comes from an intriguing study, carried out in Greece, which set out to measure what happened when people increased their consumption of certain types of food — including meat and vegetables.[23] The results show that an increase in taking spinach, beets, cabbage or lettuce actually *decreases* your chance of contracting colo-rectal cancer. But on the other hand, an increase in beef or lamb consumption *increases* your risk. This is what it looks like graphically:

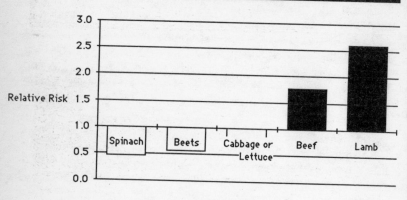

RISK OF COLO-RECTAL CANCER WITH DOUBLING IN FOOD ITEM CONSUMPTION FROM ONCE TO TWICE PER WEEK: THE GREEK STUDY

The study concludes as follows:

'The results of most of these studies appear to fall into two broad categories: those indicating that animal protein (mainly beef meat) and/or animal fat are conducive to the development of colo-rectal cancer — and those indicating that vegetables (particularly cruciferous vegetables) or, more generally, fibre-containing foods, protect against the development of this disease.'

The Last Word

For our last study, we are going to look at the results of one of the largest surveys ever undertaken.[24] In 1965, researchers in Japan began to painstakingly question over 122,000 men aged forty or more. They were monitored until 1981, by which time 30,000 of them had died, 8,000 from cancers. All of them were divided into six groups, according to their propensity to smoke, drink alcohol, eat meat, and consume fresh vegetables. Have a look at the results, and we'll discuss them after you've seen the chart:

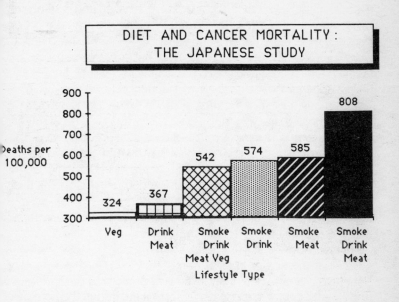

These are the important points to emerge from this enormous study:

● The safest group, on the extreme left, are those who do not eat meat, smoke, or drink alcohol, but who do eat fresh vegetables.
● The group most at risk, on the extreme right, are those who eat meat, smoke, and drink alcohol, but who do not consume fresh vegetables.

But just look at the columns in the middle. A group that shares the same lifestyle as the high risk group (meat, smoke, drink) *and also includes* fresh vegetables reduces their death-rate by one third. Although, of course, this is still twice as high as those who don't take meat, drink or smoke. So perhaps some vegetables *do* have a protective effect against cancer.

Research versus History

We have examined a great deal of material, but it is still only a small fraction of the research that has been undertaken and is still going on. It may take many years to finally establish the connection between meat consumption and cancer to everyone's satisfaction. Some people may never be convinced. But as the years go by, and the mortality correlations keep on coming in, it will be harder and harder for them not to accept the evidence.

If humans have been eating meat in some form or other for thousands of years, you may wonder why it is only recently that the connection with various forms of cancer has been spotted. This is a good question, and one which has several answers.

Firstly, we know that humans have suffered from cancer for about the same length of time that they have been eating animal flesh — the difference is that these days, modern science has allowed us to objectively demonstrate that meat is a risk factor. We never had the tools to prove this in the past.

But also, never — in the whole of human history — have humans eaten so much animal flesh as part of their diets as they do today. In neolithic times (only a short time ago in terms of the human body's evolution) meat comprised only a fraction of the total diet. But today, the average Westernized household consumes nearly *ten pounds* of meat every week. Just imagine how large that is — it's the size of a human baby. Our bodies have never had to exist on such an intensive diet. We are performing a new experiment with them, and it's not surprising that there are some unpleasant side-effects. Additionally of course, the *type* and *quality* of meat that is available today is very, very different to that which was eaten even just a century or more ago. The meat industry has seen to that.

Some Clues to the Problem

So how does meat actually *cause* cancer? There is much on-going research into this but, even so, it may be several decades before any firm conclusions are reached. The epidemiological process is always a slow one. And there are many extremely powerful vested interests who, frankly, have no desire for the consumer to know all the facts. Nevertheless, some basic connections have already been made.

It is well-known, for example, that charcoal-grilled steak contains significantly large quantities of a powerful carcinogen, benzopyrene. In just one kilogram of steak there is as much benzopyrene as in the smoke from *six hundred* cigarettes.

It is also well-known that pork products contain nitrites, which are often added to prolong shelf-life and give a pink colour to the meat. But the problem with nitrites is that they combine with other substances in the human body to form nitrosamines which are the most powerful nervous system carcinogens yet discovered. These are just some of the better-known cancer-promoting agents found in meat.

Surely, you may wonder, such carcinogenic substances can't be *allowed* to contaminate the food that much of the public eats? Someone, somewhere, must control what's permitted to be added, and regulate the system? In theory, of course, someone *is* reponsible. But in practice, it just doesn't seem to work out. In the United Kingdom, lack of manpower (and it seems, the willpower) together with unnecessary restrictions on freedom of information together conspire to keep us in a state of ignorance.

And even in the United States, where much more information may be made public, the situation doesn't seem to be any better. Just recently, a Congressional report into the mighty Food and Drug Administration concluded that its inadequate food monitoring procedures posed a 'grave threat' to the health of consumers, singling out beef and pork for particular condemnation. They found farmers using literally thousands of animal drugs and feed supplements on their meat animal that had *never* been approved for use — and some of which had actually been proven scientifically to be cancer-causing. Said Congressman Ted Weiss, Chairman of the Inquiry:

> The law requires and consumers deserve far more public health protection than the agency has provided. The Food and Drug Administration has repeatedly put what it perceives are interests of veterinarians and the livestock industry ahead of its legal obligation to protect consumers. [25]

Cancer — the Big Unanswered Question

There is one more connection between human cancer and meat consumption that you ought to be aware of. At the moment, it has not been fully and finally proven, because it is ethically unacceptable for scientists to try and induce cancers in human populations for experimental purposes. Nevertheless, the circumstancial evidence is strong enough to allow us to ask the question:

'Can you get cancer from eating cancerous meat?'

The connection is really very simple. First — we know that some meat producing animals (especially cows and chickens) suffer from tumours and cancers. Second — we know that cancer can be transmitted by virus, from one animal to another, and indeed from one species to another. Third — cancerous and tumourous meat is not all removed at the slaughterhouse, and may quite easily find its way to the butcher's shop. The chances are that, if you eat meat, sooner or later you will eat part of an animal that either has cancer or has been exposed to a virus that can cause cancer. It is difficult to quantify the risk you would be running by eating tumourous meat (especially since cancers can take many years to surface), but it is a problem you should be aware of.

The first clue that cancer could be transmitted by a virus came as far back as 1908, when two investigators showed they could transmit leukaemia from one chicken to another. Again, in 1911, experiments showed that solid lumps of tumour, taken from one chicken and implanted into another, would infect the second chicken with a cancerous growth. But despite this early evidence, it took many more years for most scientists to publicly admit that cancer _could_ be caused and/or transmitted by a virus. More recently, it has been shown that substances with carcinogenic properties can somehow 'awaken' viruses in one animal, which can then be passed on to another. One experiment demonstrated this by using X-rays to cause leukaemia in a mouse. A virus was then produced in the mouse's leukaemic cells, which could then infect other mice with leukaemia. Here is a summary of the evidence currently available that supports the cancer/meat connection:

● Viruses are currently implicated in sixty per cent of _all_ human infections. It has gradually been proven that a considerable number of viruses can be passed from animals to humans — some examples being rabies, yellow fever, cow pox and encephalitis. Additionally, some viruses may only produce cancer in humans, not animals, and be very slow acting.

● Marek's disease (a scourge amongst chickens) is caused by a Herpes virus. A recent scientific report establised that 'there is a strong association between the possession of antibodies to Herpes simplex virus (HSV) type 2 and cervical carcinoma of women.'[26]

● In Africa, it has been shown that a certain type of cancer only occurs in humans in low-altitude, high-temperature, high-rainfall regions that tend to harbour both African clawed frogs and mosquitos. The cancer probably originates in the frogs, and is transferred to man via mosquito bite, thus showing that inter-species virus transmission may be possible.[27]

● The animal/human/virus transmission process may work the other way round, as well. It has been observed that healthy dogs who come into contact with children with leukaemia subsequently have a type C virus in their blood plasma.[27]

● One study has shown that a 'helper virus' can form an association with another relatively harmless one, and in the process produce a virus that can induce cancer. One such virus (the Rous sarcoma virus) occurs in chickens. There is the possibility that such a virus may enter the human body and convert harmless human viruses into killers[27]

● In one ethically-questionable experiment, humans already suffering from advanced cancer were inocculated with a virus that was known to cause cancer amongst monkeys. The patients all developed the same tumours as the monkeys. A laboratory worker also inocculated himself by accident, and developed a tumour.[26]

● Cows, chickens and turkeys are known to suffer from 'leucosis', a form of cancer that is known to be produced by a virus. Leucosis produces multiple tumours, and sometimes goes on to produce leukaemia in the animals too. It has been shown that virus-like particles exist in the milk taken from herds of cows where there is a high incidence of leucosis.[28]

● It has been shown in experiments that Bovine Leukaemia Virus (the virus that causes leucosis in cattle) can survive and replicate itself when placed in a human culture.[29]

● In an experiment on chimpanzees, they were fed from birth on milk taken from cows known to be infected with Bovine Leukaemia Virus. They died from leukaemia.[30]

● A study of mortality from leukaemia and Hodgkin's disease amongst vets has shown that they run a significantly higher risk of dying from lymphoid cancer than the norm. These vets were in clinical practice, in close contact with food-producing animals, and the authors of the report suggested that a viral cause may be responsible.[31]

● A statistical analysis of human deaths from leukaemia in Nebraska showed that, in men aged between forty and sixty years, the mortality rate was twice as high amongst men with regular contact with cattle than the norm.[32]

● Further studies have shown a strong relationship between farm animal contact and deaths from leukaemia, with poultry farmers particularly at risk:[33] in Poland it was shown that leukaemia was significantly more common in people having regular contact with animals, such as farmers, butchers, and tanners,[34] and in Minnesota an investigation conducted amongst leukaemia sufferers showed that a higher than expected number of them were farmers having regular contact with animals.[35]

● Another report investigated an outbreak of leucosis amongst cows in a dairy farm in the United States, and found that over a ten year period two farm employees and two farm neighbours all developed leukaemia of the same type.[36]

● Extensive experimental work with the viruses that cause leucosis in poultry has proven that they can be transmitted from chickens to other animals, including rats, mice, hamsters, guinea pigs, rabbits, dogs, and monkeys. It has also been shown that these viruses can affect human cells kept in experimental cultures.[37,38,39]

What does all this evidence mean? I would simply suggest that it indicates that much more scientific work needs to be undertaken on this worrying subject. In the mean time, there is little doubt that at last some of the meat eaten today comes from animals that are suffering from some form of cancer.

Of course, meat is supposed to be inspected at the slaughter-house, so I asked one veterinary surgeon with responsibility for meat inspection to tell me what regulations, if any, applied to tumourous carcasses. He told me that meat hygiene regulations were difficult to enforce, particularly with regard to poultry.

'It's the feeling of many Official Veterinary Surgeons that poultry inspection standards are being whittled away,' he told me. 'Until we joined the EEC, the inspection was pretty minimal in any case. Now, the standards are dropping again. For example, if you're someone who rears and kills your own birds (and many people do), then there's no requirement for any inspection at all.'

'What about tumours and other cancers in meat?' I asked him. He pulled out his file concerning the Meat Inspection Regulations. 'It's an interesting situation', he said. 'If a carcass contains just one tumour, then it would be cut out of the carcass and condemned. But the rest of the carcass would be passed.'

'So no-one would ever know that the animal had cancer?' I enquired. 'That's right', he said. 'But if the carcass contains two or more tumours, then the whole carcass would be condemned. It could then go for pet food. Although sometimes condemned meat has a habit of turning up as fit for human consumption.'

'I understand that a meat inspector on a poultry line has three to five seconds to examine each bird and judge whether it's healthy,' I said. 'Is that sufficient time to give it a clean bill of health, free from tumours?'

The vet smiled and told me that, even with his experience, he couldn't perform an autopsy *that* quickly.

The Verdict

In this chapter we have examined some of the relationships between meat consumption and the occurrence of certain forms of cancer, principally breast cancer, colon cancer, prostate cancer, and other intestinal cancers. But there is also a growing body of evidence that meat eating may relate to other forms of cancers as well.

Recent research into cancer of the ovaries has established a meat connection. 'There was a significant trend towards increasing risk for ovarian cancer with increasing animal fat consumption,' said one study, and it found that women who consume the most animal fat in their diet run *double* the risk of contracting ovarian cancer when compared to those who consume the least.[40]

Yet another study concluded that men who heavily consume animal products run nearly *four times* the risk of contracting fatal cancer of the prostate, when compared with those who do not consume such large quantities.[41]

Even more disturbing evidence is also coming to light concerning the development of brain tumours in young children. A study has indicated that a significant risk factor is the amount of contact that the mother may have had with nitrosamines — and this is directly related to maternal consumption of cured meats.[42]

At the same time as the case against meat is looking increasingly grim, the case in favour of a higher fresh fruit and vegetable intake is looking better and better. In studies, Vitamins C, A and E have all been shown to inhibit cancer growth. So have such exotically-named substances as indoles, coumarins, aromatic isothiocyanates, flavones, phenols, and plant sterols — and yes, they're all found in the vegetable kingdom.

Studies have also shown that cancer patients frequently experience sudden changes in their dietary preferences — away from fatty meats, towards fresher things. 'Foods in the classes of red meats, white meat, fish or poultry, and high protein foods were rated significantly less pleasant by patients with cancer,' said one study. 'This aversion was apparently most marked for red meats . . . Roast beef had the largest percentage, forty-four per cent, of reported taste change.'[43] It's easy to speculate, of course. But could it just be that their bodies are trying to tell them something?

So how long will it take for our officials, our governments, and our food producers to take the lead, and actually *encourage* us to stop eating suspect foods, and start eating healthily? Well, it may take for ever. The American Dietetic Association came the closest that perhaps any official body has ever come to doing this when it made this official statement:

> The American Dietetic Association recognizes that a growing body of scientific evidence supports a positive relationship between the consumption of a plant-based diet and the prevention of certain diseases.[40]

But for now, as they say, it's over to you. Because if you don't take the right decisions to look after your own health, then no-one else is going to.

REFERENCES

1. 'Cancer Statistics', Office of Population Censuses and Surveys, Cancer Research Campaign, Studies on Medical and Population Subjects No. 43, HMSO 1981.
2. Higson J. Muir CS. 'Environmental Carcinogenesis', J. Natl Cancer Inst. 1979; 63: 1291-8, and others.
3. *The Causes of Cancer*, R. Doll and R. Peto, Oxford Medical Publications, 1981.

4. 'Diet and Cardiovascular Disease', COMA report (Committee on Medical Aspects of Food Policy), DHSS 1984.

5. *Eastern Daily Press* 20 February 1984.

6. Quoted in 'In Defence of the British Pork Pie', R. Collins, *The Guardian* 13 January 1986.

7. *Eastern Daily Press*, 3 December 1984.

8. *Eastern Daily Press*, 4 December 1984.

9. *Staffordshire Newsletter*, 17 May 1985.

10. 'Gastrointestinal Cancer and Nutrition', O. Gregor, R. Toman, F. Prusova, Gut 10 (12): 1031-1034.

11. Quoted in *Time*, 18 November 1985.

12. For example, see 'Dietary Factors Associated with Death-Rates from certain Neoplasms in Man'. A. J. Lea, *The Lancet*, 6 August 1966.

13. 'Environmental Factors of Cancer of the Colon and Rectum', Ernest L. Wynder, Takao Shigematsu, *Cancer*, September 1967, Vol 20, no9, p. 1528.

14. From data in 'Role of Life-style and Dietary habits in Risk of Cancer among Seventh-day Adventists', Roland L. Phillips, *Cancer Research*, 35, 3513-3522, November 1975.

15. Quoted in 'Role of Life-style and Dietary habits in Risk of Cancer among Seventh-day Adventists', Roland L. Phillips, *Cancer Research*, 35, 3513-3522, November 1975 from data in 'Death from Respiratory Disease among Seventh-day Adventist Men', F. R. Lemon, R. T. Walden, J.Am.Med.Assoc. 189:117-126, 1966 and 'Cancer of the Lung and Mouth in Seventh-day Adventists', F. R. Lemon, R. T. Walden, R. W. Woods, *Cancer*, 17:486-497, 1964.

16. 'Association of Meat and Coffee Use with Cancers of the Large Bowel, Breast and Prostate among Seventh Day Adventists: Preliminary Results', Roland L. Phillips, David A. Snowdon; *Cancer Research*, 43:2403-2408, May 1983.

17. 'Mortality among Japanese Zen Priests', M. Ogatu, M. Ikeda, M. Kuratsune, *Journal of Epidemiology and Community Health*, 1984,38,161-166.

18. 'Diet as an Etiological Factor in the Development of Cancers of the Colon and Rectum', M. A. Howell, J. *Chron.Dis.*, 1975,28,67-80.

19. 'Association Between Dietary Changes and Mortality Rates: Israel 1949-1977; a Trend-Free Regression Model', A. Palgi, *American Journal of Clinical Nutrition*, 34, August 1981, pp 1569-1583.

20. 'Dietary Factors and Breast Cancer Risk', J. H. Lubin, P. E. Burns, W. J. Blot, R. G. Ziegler, A. W. Lees, J. F. Fraumeni, *Int. J. Cancer*, 28, 685-689, 1981.

21. 'Nutrient Intakes in Relation to Cancer Incidence in Hawaii', L. N. Kolonel, J. H. Hankin, J. Lee, S. Y. Chu, A. M. Y. Nomura, M. Ward Hines, Br. J. Cancer 1981 44,332.

22. 'Epidemiological Correlations Between Diet and Cancer Frequency', P. Correa, Cancer Research, 41, 3685-3690.

23. 'Diet and Colo-Rectal Cancer: A Case-Control Study in Greece', O. Manousos, N. E. Day, D. Trichopoulos, F. Gerovassilis, A. Tzonou, Int. J. Cancer, 32,1-5 1983.

24. Dr. Takeshi Hirayama, National Cancer Research Institute, Tokyo.

25. New York Times, 13 January 1986.

26. 'Recent advances in viral zoonoses', Rajinder Jerath, Int. J. Zoonoses, 6;49-60, 1979.

27. 'Virus Cancer Research,' No 1130, 1968 Washington DC National Cancer Institute.

28. 'Virus-like Particles in Cow's Milk from a Herd with a High Incidence of Lymphosarcoma,' R. M. Dutcher, E. P. Larkin, R. R. Marshak, JNCI, 33, 1055-1064.

29. 'Induction of Syncytia by the Bovine C-type Leukaemia Virus,' C. A. Diglio, J. F. Ferrer, Cancer Research, 36:1056-1067.

30. 'Erythroleukaemia in Two infant Chimpanzees fed milk from Cows naturally infected with the Bovine C-type Virus,' H. M. McClure, M. E. Keeling, R. P. Custer, R. R. Marshak, D. A. Abt, J. F. Ferrer, Cancer Research, 34:2745-2757.

31. 'Cancer and other causes of death among US Veterinarians 1966-1977,' A. Blair, H. M. Hayes, International Journal of Cancer, 25:181-185.

32. 'Food-born viruses and malignant hemopoietic diseases,' H. M. Lemon, Bact. Rev., 28:490-492.

33. 'Leukaemia and multiple myeloma in farmers,' S. Milham, American Journal of Epidemiology, 94:307-310.

34. 'Leukaemia in humans and animals in the light of epidemiological studies with reference to problems of its prevention,' J. Aleksandrowicz, Acta Med. Polona, 9:217-230.

35. 'Leukaemia in Olmsted county, Minnesota, 1965-1974,' A. Linos, R. A. Kyle, L. R. Elveback, L. T. Kurland, Mayo Clin. Proc., 53:714-718.

36. 'Human leukaemia: genetic and environmental clusters,' C. W. Heath, Bibl. Haematol, 36:649-653.

37. Oncogenic Viruses, L. Gross, 2nd ed., Pergamon Press, New York, 1970.

38. 'Presence of particles with the morphology of viruses of the avian leukosis complex in meningeal tumours induced in dogs by Rous

sarcoma virus', G. F. Robotti, *Virology*, 24:686.

39. 'Avian tumour viruses', P. K. Vogt, *Adv. Virus Res.*, 7:293.

40. 'Dietary animal fat in relation to Ovarian cancer risk', D. W. Cramer, W. R. Welch, G. B. Hutchinson, W. Willett, R. E. Scully, *Obstetrics and Gynaecology*, Vol 63, No 6 June 1984.

41. 'Diet, Obesity and Risk of fatal prostate cancer', D. A. Snowdon, R. L. Phillips, W. Choi, *American Journal of Epidemiology*, 1984; 120:244-50.

42. 'N-Nitroso Compounds and childhood brain tumours: A case-control study', S. Preston-Martin, M. C. Yu, B. Benton, B. E. Henderson, *Cancer Research* Vol 42;5240-5245, December 1982.

43. 'Food Preferences of patients with cancer', Z. M. Vickers, S. S. Nielsen, A. Theologides, *Journal of the American Dietetic Association*, Vol 79, October 1981.

44. 'Position paper on the vegetarian approach to eating', *Journal of the American Dietetic Association*, Vol 77, July 1980.

4

Breaking Free!

At this point you may want some practical advice about kicking the flesh food habit. People who've already stopped eating meat are usually completely puzzled when anyone asks them: 'How do you go about cutting it out?' You see, they no longer even think about it. For most people, it quickly becomes a normal part of their lifestyle, and they just can't *imagine* how it could present a problem to anyone.

I used to think this, too. But now I know, from many letters, conversations and phone calls from anxious parents, worried husbands, and lots of other people as well, that cutting out meat from your diet can *seem* to be an almost impossible achievement. Impossible, that is, until you do it.

Don't Panic!

The first thing to do is to *stop worrying*! You're absolutely certain to have many different questions going through your mind, such as 'Where do I get my protein from?' 'What do I replace meat with?' 'Can I eat fish?' and so on . . . Well, you'll find the answers to most of the commonest questions right here in this book. But at this stage, the most important thing is not to panic, and to plan the transition so that it suits *you*. Speak to other people who've made the break, by all means, but don't forget that what suits one person may not be right for *you*. That's really the key. Because, maybe for the first time in your entire life, you're going to take full control over the food you eat.

The Revolution Starts Here

One of life's biggest con-tricks is to make us believe that we choose the food we eat for ourselves. Nothing could be further from the truth. You may *think* that your taste preferences reflect your own likes and dislikes, but in all probability they owe more to your parents than they really do to you. As human infants, we are more dependent upon our parents and more vulnerable over a far greater period of time than any other species on the face of the Earth. It takes us years to achieve the same degree of control over even the most basic of our activities that the young of other species manage to achieve in a matter of months or even weeks.

Year after year, we rely upon adults to take most of our simple everyday decisions for us. Now, biologically speaking, this works out very well because we have a lot more growing to do than most other species do, and while we're doing all this growing we need the protection that parents can give us.

But parents give you more than just protection. They pass on to you their own values and beliefs, to the extent that by the time you're old enough to take informed decisions for yourself, you've acquired a whole set of inherited likes, dislikes and habits that, by sheer force of repetition, you've grown to regard as your own. Habits such as the way you eat, for example. And what you eat, and indeed, what you think about what you eat. All these habits have been largely pre-determined for you. Other people have taken these decisions, because you weren't able to at the time. But you *are* able to now.

Meat Hooked?

The difficult thing with meat is that, just like tobacco and some other drugs, although you may not enjoy it at the beginning, your taste buds get hooked on its fatty, salty flavour quite quickly. Man is not the only animal to respond to meat like this — chimpanzees (whose diets are naturally meat-free) will behave in a similar way. A chimp who has tasted carrion flesh a few times will progress to hunting and killing for himself, sometimes even committing acts of cannibalism and infanticide against his own species. Gorillas are also naturally gentle and non-meat eating, but when captive ones in zoos have been forcibly fed a meat diet they, too, will develop mammoth carnivorous appetites — the more they eat, the more they must have. These behavioural changes are also accompanied by physical changes in their digestive system whereby the ciliate protozoa (useful micro-organisms we all need) in their intestines which would normally help to digest the fibre in their natural diet disappear. So returning to plant food isn't very easy for them.

It isn't so strange, then, that young humans also become accustomed to the taste of meat, and grow up to consider large quantities of it to be an indispensible part of their diet. However, what has really happened is that we have been 'taught' to eat meat, taught to regard its taste as palatable, and taught to consider it (if, indeed, we think about it at all) as a perfectly normal part of our diet. Many young children instinctively resist eating meat — perhaps you did, too. But by the time you were old enough to think objectively about the issue, you may already have been hooked.

The only chance to break into this circle is to do precisely what you're doing now — to examine the evidence, and to take an informed decision based on your own personal feelings. I seriously believe that this may be the most important decision that you've ever taken. It may be the first time that you've ever had the chance to consciously and rationally reclaim control of a crucial area of your daily activity, that has, until now, been pre-programmed by a pattern of behaviour that someone else decided upon several decades ago. It's a great opportunity to get things *right!*

Making the Break

So what happens? Do you come home at 6 o'clock one Friday evening and have a nut cutlet instead of a lamb cutlet? Do you have to sign a pledge that meat will never pass your lips again? Or do you just do it in private, with consenting adults? Here are some ideas for making the break that I know have worked very well with other people. But do remember that fundamentally it's *your* decision — you're trying to find what genuinely suits *you*. So you should take everything that follows as suggestions, not as firm rules.

Method One: The Cut-Back

This may be useful if you *want* to kick the meat habit, but are worried that you wouldn't know where to start. Basically, you should aim to reduce your meat intake by about fifty per cent per week. For example, if you regularly eat meat at two meals a day, cut this back during the first week to just one meal a day. Then, for the second week, cut it back again to one meal every other day. The third week you probably won't eat more than a couple of meat meals in total. And the fourth week you'll be free. This gradual process of cutting back gives you the chance to spread the transition over several weeks, and so allows you to experiment with lots of new recipes, while being able to fall back on meat if you get desperate! It sometimes helps to deliberately switch the type of meat you'd normally eat to something you dislike. So if you dislike mutton, for example, make sure that any meat you eat is mutton. This will help your body to reinforce the decision you've made. The disadvantage with this method is that it can take a lot of will power to get to the 'no-meat' stage. So you could try combining the first week or two of this method with one of the others.

Method Two: The Green-Out

This is a fairly dramatic technique that will appeal to those people who want to create a clear, precise point in their lives that may represent a kind of personal watershed for them. It also has quite a profound effect on your body, so you should check with your doctor if your health may raise problems.

What you do is to eat a completely raw diet for seven to ten days.

Nothing — absolutely nothing — that has been cooked, processed or preserved is allowed down! Meat, of course, is right out. So is cheese, although you could eat a raw egg if you could stomach it (too frequent use of raw eggs could lead to a biotin deficiency, so don't overdose!). Similarly, bread, biscuits, jams, butter, tea, coffee, alcohol, and tinned food are all absolutely out. However, the diet, must contain lots of fresh fruit and vegetables — there is no limit to the quantity, eat as much as you can take. Aim to buy organic vegetables, if at all possible. Don't overlook nuts and seeds, and try making salad dressings using only cold-pressed oils and lemon juice for a delicious dressing. In practice, you'll find it very difficult to over-eat on raw food. Although you'll be taking in lots of vitamins from all this fresh food, it might be a good idea to supplement your diet with a good multi-vitamin pill that includes calcium and zinc (generally, I'm firmly against them because you should get your nourishment from a well-balanced diet, but they'll help at least psychologically on this occasion).

During this period all sorts of things may start to happen. You may feel wonderfully elated or (very rarely) rather depressed. Your body may start to feel lighter and younger. On the other hand, you may very well have some kind of 'deferred reaction' — you may get spots and pimples, a bad headache, or diarrhoea (don't be surprised if you do, because your intestinal micro-flora is changing!). Stick with it, because it won't last very long, and you'll feel much better when you've been through it. After seven to ten days, you can start to add some cooked food, which you've been reading about in the meantime. You'll also find that your tastes have started to change. You will almost certainly have developed an appreciation for fresh food, and a healthy desire to eat something fresh at least once a day. And then you won't look back! You will have made the break, given your body a thorough detoxification, and started to set the pattern for a better, healthier life.

Method Three: The Switcheroo

I can't wholeheartedly recommend this method, but I know that

many people have, almost by default, used it. Basically, all that'
involved is substituting a non-meat product for meat, on ever
occasion a recipe calls for meat.

The range of meat replacement products is getting better all the
time, and finding an acceptable substitute shouldn't be a problem
You should be able to purchase textured vegetable protein (tvp
from any health food shop, in a wide variety of flavourings and
textures. There are also many commercial mixtures, such a
sausages, burger mixes, pâtes, etc., that are all 100 per cent non
meat, and advertised as such. Most health food stores are full c
them, although some may be rather expensive. The cheapes
substitute is probably to purchase loose tvp granules (unflavoured
and experiment with flavourings that please you. Some to try are
yeast extract, tamari (a kind of soya sauce), or even an ordinar
commercial gravy mixture (surprisingly, not all of them actuall
contain meat!). You may also consider substituting meat with
seafood, cheese, eggs and other dairy produce, but try to avoid
high fat products.

I think this method can be useful in situations where the coo
is totally unfamiliar with anything other than meat cookery, such
as an older mother having to cater for a son or daughter who'
given up meat. The reason I don't like it too much is because i
doesn't encourage you to *think* about your diet, which is one c
the great opportunities that cutting out meat gives you. The
tendency is just to go on eating in the same old way — which ma
not be very healthy. It seems a shame to waste such a great chance

Breaking the News

This, too, can create a lot of problems for people, although there'
no reason why it should. There seem to be two sorts of problems
One is the 'Oh-My-God-How-Are-You-Going-To-Survive' reaction, tha
typically comes from over-worried friends and relatives. The othe
is the 'Oh-My-God-What-Am-I-Going-To-Cook' reaction from the
cook. Both can verge on the hysterical, so try to disarm them earl
on.

If we take the first reaction, which mainly comes from family or friends, as basically being a sign of well-meaning concern, then it shouldn't upset you too much. Maybe they can't imagine what you're going to exist on when you quit meat, and they're obviously expecting you to shrivel up and die at any moment. In a word, they're ignorant. So enlighten them! Lend them this book, talk to them about it *ad nauseam*, try to get them involved. Tell them about famous people such as Leonardo Da Vinci, Voltaire, George Bernard Shaw, and all the many others who existed without eating flesh. If there's a good wholefood restaurant nearby, suggest that you all go out and have a meal together. Don't try to sell them the idea if they're not ready for it, but do try to reassure them, which is all that's really needed.

The second reaction is usually found among mothers who find they've suddenly got to cope with a meat-free menu. Not surprisingly, they feel as if they've been dropped in the deep end. The best advice here is to discuss the situation with them as early as you can. Tell them that more and more people are finding a better, healthier way of eating, and for a variety of reasons you'd like to try it too. You'll probably have to lead the way by obtaining a few *simple* recipe books, and also by doing your fair share of kitchen work. Providing you take it slowly and don't panic them, you'll probably find that they are extremely interested in what you're doing, and may try it as well.

Keep On Truckin'

Once you get started, you won't want to stop. You may well notice that other — apparently unconnected — aspects of your life will change for the better, too. I'm not sure how or why this happens, but I do know that many people — perhaps the majority — experience a real increase in the quality of their own lives. Sometimes, it can be a very profound change indeed, and can shape a person's future in an entirely new and unexpected way. You may find your attitudes changing, or opening up. I compare it to a conveyor belt, that you've somehow managed to activate. It doesn't matter where you get on, it can still take you a bit further along. That's all I can really tell you about it, because the experience is one that is uniquely personal. If you recognize this phenomenon in *your* life, don't fight it — see where it leads . . .

A Few Good Books . . .

There has been such an explosion of interest in meat-free cookery recently that many publishers have quickly rushed out books designed to cash in on the market. Some of them are genuinely useful, but some of them are dreary and not very enticing. So here are a few recipe books that I can wholeheartedly recommend from personal experience:

The Farm Vegetarian Cookbook,
Edited by Louise Hagler, The Book Publishing Company (United States, imported into Britain by Thorsons).

Not very easy to find in every bookshop, but worth searching out or ordering specially. This has been my favourite general-purpose cookbook for some time. Its recipes don't even use eggs, milk or any dairy produce, but despite that, each one I've tried is a real winner. You won't find many familiar recipe names here and may feel rather lost initially, particularly if you're used to a conventional cookbook, so it might be too much to take all at once. It's got some good suggestions featuring tvp, and most of them are very suitable for children. It also gives you the clearest, no-fuss guide to making your own tofu that I've found. Many recipes are soya bean based, since the book is basically a compilation of recipes submitted by members of a community called 'The Farm,' who live on 1,750 acres in Tennessee and grow their own soya crop. Reading this book will give you a healthy respect for the incredibly versatile and bountiful soya bean. As a result, I bought a sack of beans (45 kilograms), which has now provided us with hundreds of tasty and nutritious meals, at a ridiculously low cost — and there are still plenty left! The book also includes sections on Mexican food, gluten, tempeh, soya milk and yogurt, yuba, breads, cereals and sweets. My particular favourites are Barbeque Beans, Ellen's Good for Ya Noodle Soup, Tofu Spinach Pie, Granola, and Soysages.

The Vegetarian Epicure,
Anna Thomas, Vintage Books, New York.

Also available in the U.K. as a Penguin edition, but unfortunately lacking the size, beautiful design, and 'feel' of the American edition, which you should get for preference. This is much more straightforward fare, and perhaps easier for a newcomer to come to terms with. It's a very friendly book, contains 262 recipes with complete menu suggestions, and it was obviously written as a labour of love. Most of the recipes are easy to prepare, and include such tasties as Lentil Soup Creole, Gazpacho, a good selection of multi-purpose sauces, Spanakopit, some truly wonderful pasta dishes, some 'holiday' recipes, and much else besides to suit almost everyone.

Indian Vegetarian Cooking,
Michael Pandya, Thorsons.

You either love or loathe Indian cooking, and if (like me) you love it, then this book is simply wonderful. If you don't happen to like Indian food, the book just might manage to tempt you! It's important to realize that there is virtually no connection between *real* Indian cookery and the sort of food that is served up at most so-called Indian restarants and take-aways. If you've been lucky enough to go to India, or if you've ever had a meal prepared for you by an Indian family, you'll know what I mean. This book has the authentic taste of India in it, which it shows you how to re-create in your own kitchen. And there's a particular fascination in collecting and mixing your own spices (hint — this seems to appeal to many men). It tells you what sort of spices to buy and how to combine them, and lists recipes from all over India, with widely differing styles. Like anything new, you've got to work your way into it, and there may be one or two things that don't suit you. But the simple and quick recipe for *dhuli masoor dhal* (washed lentils) is a classic among classics, being the best I've ever tasted, and putting the thin, watery tasteless substance most Indian restaurants serve as *dal* to shame. It includes complete sections on soups and hot drinks, Indian bread dishes, rice, pulses and legumes, curries, sauces, relishes and pickles, savouries and Indian sweets, and cold drinks.

Laurel's Kitchen,
Laurel Robertson, Routledge and Kegan Paul.

A very comprehensive cookery book, running over 500 pages, complete with very detailed nutritional information (in fact probably more than you need to know). It was one of the earliest classics of meat-free cookery, and is written with real enthusiasm that's contagious. It's careful to take you through things stage by stage, so you can read it like a novel, from one cover to the other. There's a good discussion of most aspects of meat-free cookery, and its coverage on bread and bread making is particularly good, and interesting to read too. This is a valuable book for most people.

Let's Cook It Together!,
Peggy Brusseau, Thorsons.

I ought to disclose my personal interest right away, and tell you that this book was written by my wife, so I've got first-hand experience of every single recipe in it! It's unlike any other cookery book, because it is written for parents and children to use *together*. The aim is to make preparing the family food a shared, joyful experience. Every recipe is new, and designed to maximize the amount of fun you can have in a kitchen, while teaching the basics of good cookery skills and nutrition. Unlike some other recipe books written 'for' children, it doesn't patronize, and it can be used at almost any age. And who can resist recipes with names like 'Short, Fat and Sassy,' 'Paul Bunyan's Tears,' or 'Slugs and Snails'?

The Vegetarian Baby,
Sharon Yntema, Thorsons.

Useful advice on nutrition during pregnancy right through to the two-year-old. Written from personal experience, very reassuring and informative.

The Book Of Tofu,
William Shurtleff and Akiko Aoyagi, Autumn Press (U.S.A., distributed by Random House).

Just in case you get totally turned on by tofu, as happened to me, you might want to take things a bit further, and there's no doubt that this book will prove a treasure-chest of information, recipes and processes for you. A great source-book.

The Vegetarian Cook Book,
Doreen Keighley, Thorsons.

If it's ideas you're after, this very economical book has 400 recipes for you to choose from. Don't expect lavish illustrations or flowing prose, there's just not room. But because there are so many recipes, you're bound to find something that suits you.

Cordon Vert,
Colin Spencer, Thorsons.

If you enjoy giving dinner-parties, and are worried what will happen to your social credibility if you go meat-free, this book is very definitely for you. The author is one of Britain's top food journalists (writing a column in *The Guardian*) and he has an exquisite feeling for gourmet food. The book itself is sumptuous, as are all the recipes. He's created fifty-two stunning and complete dinner menus (so you can give a party once a week for a year without duplication), and they're divided into seasonal chapters for easy availability of ingredients. No dinner party is complete without a well-chosen selection of wines and cheeses, and Spencer's suggestions are very sound.

5

Eating Your Heart Out

'Never morning wore to evening,
but some heart did break'.

— Tennyson, In Memoriam

The scientist looked proud of himself as he addressed his audience. He was talking about coronary heart disease, and the audience was spellbound.

'I predict,' he said, 'it will take five or ten years for the myths now commonly held that there is a link between animal fats and heart disease to disappear.' The audience burst into applause. This is what they wanted to hear.

'We need to present meat and animal fats as part of a well balanced diet,' he continued. 'If you give up meat, it is almost certain that you will not live any longer — but it will almost certainly seem like it for those people who enjoy eating, which after all, is one of the great pleasures of life.' He permitted a smile at his own joke. 'As far as cholesterol is concerned,' he went on, 'I can safely say that the amount of cholesterol in the blood has little or no effect on heart disease.'

The scientist's audience were not disinterested parties. He was addressing a group of beef producers, and the conference was arranged by Britain's meat industry — one of many such conferences to take place recently. They go into schools, colleges, gatherings of health-care professionals, and anywhere else a body of opinion-formers may be found. They are cleverly organized, and seek to present 'impartial' scientific evidence that portrays meat as the ideal 'health' food. Perhaps some people even believe them.

Another scientist — this time paid to come to Britain by the Milk Marketing Board — was recently flown over specially to utter these immortal words: 'I'm confident there is no data showing high-fat diets cause heart disease.' His words were widely reported.

A major sausage maker produces a leaflet all about sausages that is circulated to Britain's schoolchildren. The leaflet tells them about the wonderful protein in sausages 'and Vitamin B^1, and thiamin.' It even gives a complete nutritional analysis of an average sausage meal, including protein, calcium, fibre, vitamin C, and lots more. But what of fat? The leaflet doesn't even *mention* the word, not once. It's as if fat doesn't exist. Their boss says: 'The great British banger is here to stay. Forget the non-fat food fad and the vegetarian vogue, we are still sticking to sausages — children love bangers.' So what are we — and our children — to believe?

The facts — the real facts — are pretty clear. Some of the more important studies that connect diet with heart disease are presented to you in this chapter. Unfortunately, this is one of the few places that you'll easily find them.

The Risk of Coronary Heart Disease

Today, just like every other day in the United Kingdom, about 930 people will die from some disease of the heart and circulatory system. That's one person every one and a half minutes. Or the equivalent of wiping out an entire metropolitan borough the size of Coventry, every year. In fact, of the 630,000 people who die each year in the United Kingdom, over half of them will die from a circulatory disease. It's the biggest single cause of death.

And yet, a very large number of people do *not* die immediately. The lives of those people who linger on are rapidly changed beyond all recognition. After a lifetime of activity, they may suddenly have to get used to being incapacitated. Depression and worry is commonplace, not least over family finances. The quality of life almost inevitably deteriorates. And the increased risk of suffering another, perhaps fatal, heart attack is always present.

What is a Heart Attack?

In the fifth century B.C. the Greek doctor Hippocrates noticed that obese people were more likely to crumple up and die suddenly, but he couldn't explain why. Another clue emerged when Leonardo da Vinci described finding plaque-like deposits in the arteries of corpses he was dissecting during the course of his anatomical experiments. But it wasn't until 1912 that the first clinical observation of a coronary thrombosis, or blockage, was described, by Chicago physician James Herrick. We now know that the plaque-like material that Leonardo found is none other than cholesterol. And we also know that, strictly speaking, it's not the thrombosis (or blockage) itself that is usually the cause of death in a myocardial infarction — it is the ensuing reduced flow of blood, that directly causes a part of the heart muscle to die.

Here's the Terminology . . .

Angina Pectoris is often a warning sign that there is severe underlying heart disease. There is a deep-seated pain behind the breast-bone, which can radiate all the way down the left arm. The victim may feel extremely anxious, experience palpitations, or feel strangulation. It is often induced by physical or emotional stress. Angina may develop into a heart attack, or sometimes it may go into remission.

Arteriosclerosis is the term that is used to describe any disease which 'hardens' the arteries, so making it difficult or impossible for the blood to flow through them.

Atherosclerosis is quite simply the most common type of arteriosclerosis. It involves the creation of fatty deposits (mainly cholesterol) in the lining of the arteries thus restricting the blood flow. Although we're primarily concerned in this section with atherosclerosis as it affects the heart, it is important to realize that this is not the only target area of the body. Atherosclerosis of the arteries of the brain, for example, will cause a stroke.

Ischemic Heart Disease (I.H.D.) is the general term to describe any disease that results in a restriction of the blood flow to the heart. It's the same as coronary heart disease (also abbreviated to C.H.D.).

A *Myocardial Infarction* is what we usually think of as a heart attack. The walls of the heart muscle are called the myocardium, and when the blood can no longer reach the myocardium, that part of the heart will die. In forty per cent of all myocardial infarctions, the victim is completely unaware of any previous symptoms. He may experience intense pain, like a vice gripping his chest, shortness of breath, cold sweat, and fear of impending death. The attack may frequently be repeated within the hour.

Serum is the word used to describe the liquid portion of the blood which does not contain red cells, white cells or clotting elements.

Ventricular Fibrillation can follow a heart attack, and if not quickly corrected is invariably fatal. The heart seems to lose its rhythm, it twitches instead of beating, and can no longer pump the blood around. Blood-pressure drops to zero — sudden death is imminent. Emergency treatment in hospital involves electric shock treatment through electrodes positioned on the chest.

How Does Heart Disease Happen?

We know for sure that it starts young. In the Korean war, more than seventy-seven per cent of all soldiers killed were found to have narrowed arteries, due to atherosclerosis. Their average age was twenty-two. It is likely that it first starts with a small injury to the lining of an artery, caused by a virus, chemicals in cigarette smoke, high blood-pressure, or injury.

In the normal course of events, this small damage would be quickly repaired by the body. But sometimes, the body's maintenance men get the wrong signals. Then, instead of smoothing over the damage, the artery lining begins to swell, and the underlying muscle cells start to poke through. Large white blood cells settle on the spot, and start to extract cholesterol from the blood. The cells eventually become so engorged that they burst — but this just makes things worse, and even more white blood cells are attracted to the site. The accumulating cholesterol may serve as a seed to precipitate yet more cholesterol out of the blood. Slowly, the artery becomes more and more blocked, and the odds get shorter and shorter . . .

So what can we do about it? Is coronary heart disease simply an inevitable consequence of ageing, as some people have suggested? Or can we start to take preventative action now? The evidence suggests that we *can* do something to protect ourselves.

The First Major Study

Two pieces of evidence seemed to indicate that we should examine our diet for a possible cause of coronary heart disease. The first was that cholesterol, which had been found as deposits in the arteries, was also present in the food most western people ate. All animals, humans included, have the capacity to manufacture cholesterol. In fact, it is essential to life, and is a necessary factor in the formation of various hormones, as well as vitamin D, and helps to metabolize other fats too. And as long ago as 1913, a Russian pathologist showed that he could produce atherosclerosis in laboratory animals who were fed cholesterol-rich diets.

But the really seminal study, that primarily established the connection between diet and heart disease, began in 1947 and involved an international co-operation of researchers in Finland, Greece, Italy, Japan, the Netherlands, the United States and Yugoslavia.[1] This is the basis for contemporary thinking about diet and heart disease, and now has near-legendary status amongst researchers in the field. The study tracked a total of 12,770 men, all aged between forty and fifty-nine when the study began, and monitored them for coronary heart disease, and also undertook extensive research into each person's lifestyle. The key information that began to emerge is shown in the chart opposite which indicates very strongly that a high intake of saturated fat was linked to a high coronary death rate.

The evidence looked compelling. Deaths from heart disease are

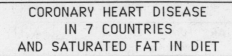

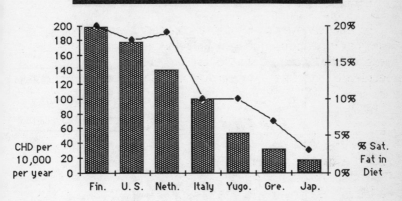

shown as columns and are plotted against the left hand axis of the graph. The intake of dietary saturated fat is shown as a line and is plotted on the right hand axis. The simple conclusion to be drawn is that the more saturated fat in a nation's diet, the greater the mortality from coronary heart disease.

The Epidemic Spreads

The researchers also found other connections. It seemed that there was also a link between the saturated fat intake and serum cholesterol — the more fat, the higher the concentration of cholesterol in the blood. This, again, supported the theory that diet and heart disease were related. There was now no time to lose. As you can see from the next chart, the death rate from coronaries was climbing higher and higher all the time. One worrying fact concerning the United Kingdom, however, should be quite obvious from this chart.[2]

In the late 1960s, the death-rate from coronaries in both Australia and the United States (both eating western-style diets) began to

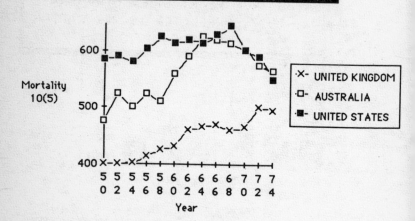

CORONARY HEART DISEASE MORTALITY
TRENDS IN MALES

Mortality
10(5)

- ·X· UNITED KINGDOM
- ·□· AUSTRALIA
- ·■· UNITED STATES

Year

tumble. But what happened in the U.K.? Quite the opposite. War-time rationing had forced the British to eat a surprisingly low-fat, healthy diet. But with the end of scarcity (and cheap butter, meat and milk), the diet — and the people — began to look sicker and sicker.

In Australia, the decline in heart disease began in 1966. Research has connected this fall with a decline in butter consumption, which started in 1952, and a decline in meat consumption, which started in 1958. In the United States, the fall in deaths from coronaries started in 1968. Again, research has connected this with a decrease in both butter and meat consumption. But, in stark contrast, both butter consumption and meat consumption kept on rising in the United Kingdom. In addition, milk, cheese and egg consumption kept on rising, and margarine consumption fell.

The picture seemed to be quite clear. Meat, as a major source of animal fat in the diet, seemed to have a distinct effect on coronary heart disease. This was confirmed again in Israel, where another important study showed that deaths from coronaries increased as the Israelis gradually took more and more meat in their diet:[3]

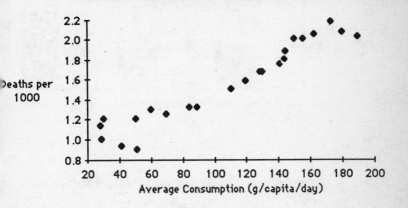

DEATHS FROM HEART DISEASE IN ISRAEL
1949-1977 CORRELATED TO PER CAPITA
MEAT CONSUMPTION

Home is Where the Heart Attacks Are

But what of the United Kingdom? While countries such as Australia and the United States were improving their own previously very high death rates, the U.K. was falling further and further behind. Coronaries today kill *forty per cent* of all men — and *thirty-eight per cent* of all women; a truly disgraceful state of affairs. Today, we have the dubious distinction of leading the world in deaths from heart disease.

There's just one bright feature in an otherwise depressing picture in this country. Studies of non-meat users indicate that they have a greatly-reduced risk of contracting coronary heart disease. The following chart says it all.[4]

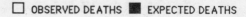

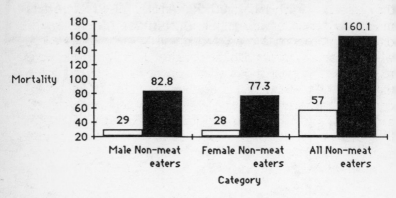

Meat's No Treat for Low-Fat Finns

Let's pause for a few moments to piece together the connections we're making. We know that cholesterol is a prime suspect in the cause of coronary heart disease. We know that there is more coronary heart disease in countries that have a diet that is high in animal (saturated) fats. So can we prove a connection between a diet rich in animal fats, and a high concentration of cholesterol in the blood?

The answer is 'Yes'. There are numerous studies that show there is just such a connection. One such study took place in Finland, a country, like the U.K., that had a very high death rate from coronaries. Except in Finland, the situation is improving. [5]

In this study, thirty families were helped to modify their diets for six weeks. The intention was not just to produce a piece of pure scientific research — it was to actually find a diet that reduced risk factors for coronary heart disease that the rest of the Finnish population could then be encouraged to adopt. So, it had to be easy to follow. Vegetable and grain products were provided free of charge, and the participants were advised to use them as much as possible. 'Hard' fats were strongly discouraged. Meat was not eliminated, but it was reduced (e.g. pork cut from forty-three grams a day to fourteen grams). The study was divided into three periods: the 'baseline', which measured the families' diets before any modification was practised; the 'intervention' period, which drastically cut back on fat consumption; and the 'switchback' period, when the families returned to their original diets. The results were remarkable. This graph shows what happened — just by modifying their diets, the people in the study brought about a very considerable drop in the saturated fat in their diet, *and also* caused a tremendous fall of twenty-three per cent in their serum cholesterol levels (the dotted line on the chart). Just as significant, too, for the scientists was a *rise* in cholesterol during the 'switchback' period — when they resumed their original diets.

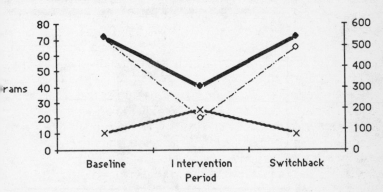

But there were other changes too. There was a significant fall in blood-pressure — generally reckoned to be a desirable thing in people at risk from coronary heart disease. The amount of polyunsaturated fats rose (due to the inclusion of more vegetables and vegetable oils), which was also beneficial. The total amount of fat dropped — from thirty-nine per cent of all calories (which is about the U.K. figure) to twenty-four per cent. And there was a twenty per cent to thirty per cent *increase* in the intake of vitamins and minerals — all those fresh vegetables. And according to the researchers, many of the Finnish families liked the taste of their new diets so much that they actually had trouble in returning to their original ones during the 'switchback' period.

Cholesterol is Something to Beef About

But this isn't the only study, by any means, that proves the connection between saturated fat and cholesterol in the blood. The next study set out to do precisely the opposite of the Finnish one — to *add* meat to the diets of people who don't normally eat it, and to observe the effects.[6] First, let's look at the chart:

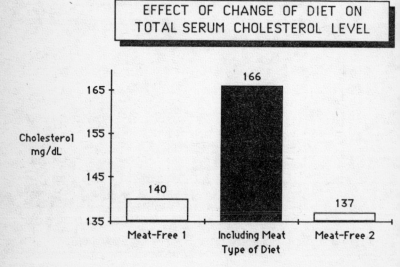

EFFECT OF CHANGE OF DIET ON TOTAL SERUM CHOLESTEROL LEVEL

A group of non-meat eaters was closely studied for two weeks, during which time their serum cholesterol was measured — see the first column on the left. Then, 250 grams of beef was added to each person's daily diet, for four weeks — and you can see from the middle column, in black, that their serum cholesterol shot up. Finally, they returned to their meatless diets, and the cholesterol again dropped to a very acceptable level. A simple experiment, but one which again shows the strong association between saturated animal fat and serum cholesterol. The researchers concluded that the change in cholesterol was equivalent to an increase from low-risk to high-risk of myocardial infarction (heart attack).

Meat is International Murder

This connection holds good on an international level, too. In countries which have a high intake of animal fat, there is a corres-

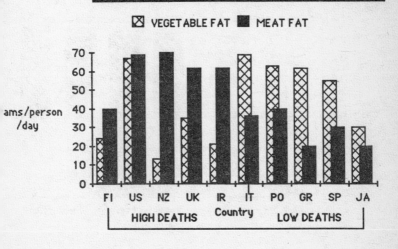

ponding high death rate from coronaries — but where plant food predominates, there are fewer mortalities. The previous chart provides a comparison of five countries with a high coronary rate (Finland), the United States, New Zealand, the United Kingdom, and Ireland) and five countries which have a low coronary mortality rate (Italy, Poland, Greece, Spain and Japan).[7]

All the countries with high mortalities are grouped on the left, and in every case meat fat consumption is very high, while vegetable fat is generally lower. On the right hand side, the countries with low death rates from coronary heart disease all have a uniformly low amount of meat fat in their diets, and instead take more vegetable fats. This is pretty strong evidence, too.

Meat the Prime Suspect

Do you remember the Seventh Day Adventists we mentioned in

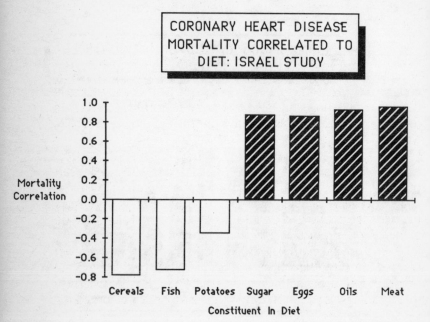

CORONARY HEART DISEASE MORTALITY CORRELATED TO DIET: ISRAEL STUDY

the section dealing with cancer? Perhaps you're wondering why no study has been undertaken using them . . . well, of course, there have been studies. And they show the same associations emerging; in the words of one report that examined 27,530 Adventists over a total of twenty-one years:

> As the frequency of meat or poultry consumption increases, so does mortality risk . . . In summary, green salad is inversely related to mortality risk, and meat and poultry are directly related to mortality risk.[8]

Other studies have also pinpointed certain areas in the diet that most strongly correlate with deaths from heart disease. One such was carried out in Israel.[3] You can see some of the results on the chart opposite. The 'good guys' are on the left hand side, and have an 'inverse correlation' with deaths from coronaries — in fact, they may even help prevent them. On the right, sugar, eggs, oils and meat are all quite strongly correlated with coronary mortality — the strongest correlation being attributed to meat.

The Crucial Question

From all the preceding evidence, it seems pretty certain that by eating a diet which is rich in animal fats we can significantly increase our risk of suffering some form of coronary heart disease. That's the bad news. But we now have to forge the final link in the chain, which may give us some good news.

The key question is this: does a *reduction* in serum cholesterol equate with a *reduction* in risk of mortality from coronary heart disease? In other words, if you *cut* your cholesterol, will you also cut your chances of dying from heart disease? Because if you can, the message is loud and clear to all of us. We could all start to do something to protect ourselves, right away.

In fact, there are many pieces of evidence that show you *can* lower your serum cholesterol level by changing your diet to eliminate or greatly reduce animal fat, and there are further studies that show that by doing this you will reduce your susceptibility to coronaries. Let's just examine a few of them.

Two mental hospitals near Helsinki, Finland, were the subject of a tightly-controlled study from 1959 to 1971.[7] The aim was to replace animal fats in the diet with vegetable fats — but without letting the patients know they were being experimented upon. For the first six years, one of the hospitals fed its patients a low animal fat, high vegetable fat diet, while the other hospital carried on as normal. Then, for the second six years, the diets were reversed, with the second hospital eating a low animal fat diet and the first hospital going back to normal. The results were very dramatic. During the experimental period, it was found that the average serum cholesterol level of the patients dropped by fifteen per cent. But even more importantly, the number of deaths due to coronary heart disease *fell by one half*. One researcher wrote:

> It is difficult to evade the conclusion that coronary heart disease is at least preventable by dietary means, but this is not to say that the problem of prevention could be completely and ultimately solved by dietary means. However, our knowledge is sufficiently extensive for its application to promote public health. It is not always judicious to wait for the final results and the irrefutable proof before taking action. Many lives could be saved and much good done by starting a little earlier. Although we do not yet have absolute proof for dietary prevention of CHD, there is strong evidence for its effectiveness, and its safety.[7]

Two further studies confirm these findings. In Oslo, two groups of men who were at risk from coronary heart disease took part in a five year experiment. One group modified their diets (by cutting back on animal fats) but the second group made no changes. After five years, the first group had lowered their average serum cholesterol by thirteen per cent. And it paid off. They had suffered an amazing forty-seven per cent *fewer* fatal and non-fatal heart attacks compared to the group who did nothing.[9]

In another study, amongst 1900 employees of the Western Electric company in the United States, there was no attempt to modify diet. Researchers simply kept records for over twenty years, and logged deaths from heart disease as they happened. Yet again, they found a positive connection between diet and serum cholesterol, and high cholesterol and mortality.[10]

The final study we'll mention again took place in the United States, and should be of tremendous importance to just about everyone. This study did not examine the effect of diet on serum cholesterol — plenty of others have already done that. Instead, researchers at the National Heart, Lung and Blood Institute at Bethesda set up a massive trial that concentrated on the beneficial effects of lowering serum cholesterol in men who were *at risk* from coronary heart disease.[11] They found 3,806 men, aged between thirty-five and fifty-nine, none of whom had actually started to develop clinical symptoms of heart disease, but all of whom showed raised cholesterol levels that put them more at risk (more than 265 mg of cholesterol per decilitre of blood, the average is 215-225 mg).

The men were randomly divided into two groups, and tracked for ten years. During this time, one group received a cholesterol-lowering drug — and the other group were given a 'placebo' to act as a comparison. At the end of the period, the group receiving the cholesterol-lowering drug showed a reduction of 8.5 per cent in serum cholesterol when compared to the other group.

Not a vast reduction, you might think. But you'd be wrong. Because even a reduction of 8.5 per cent in the serum cholesterol was enough to produce a reduction of *twenty-four per cent fewer deaths* compared to the other group.

One of the researchers went as far as to say: 'For every one per cent reduction in total cholestrol level, there is a two per cent reduction in heart disease risk.'

So here we have good, solid proof that it *is* worth trying to lower blood cholesterol levels, and that even a small reduction can appreciably reduce our chances of suffering from coronary heart disease. So what are we doing about it?

Further Fascinating Facts Featuring Fat

At this very important point, we must pause to consider the role of fat in our present-day diet. Then, in the light of the evidence we've just seen, we should be in a position to take some vital (literally life or death) decisions.

Let's think about 'fat' for a moment. What exactly does it do in our bodies? Well, its main function is to act as a storehouse for energy, which can be called upon by our muscles when they need it. The energy locked up in fat is *highly* concentrated. Energy can be measured in calories, and this chart shows how the three main constituents of our food — fat, protein and carbohydrate — compare in terms of the energy they can release:

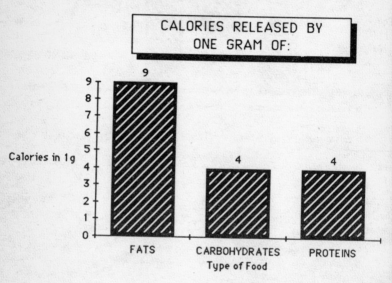

You can see that fat holds more than twice as much energy as either carbohydrate or protein. Imagine you're running a marathon. After two and a half gruelling hours running, how much fat do you think you've burnt up? In fact, you won't have used any more than a third of a pound of your body's fat. *That's* how concentrated the energy is in fat. If you're not the type to run a marathon, try walking instead. The next chart will tell you how long you've got to walk in order to burn up the energy stored in certain types of food. You may get a surprise!

That's right. You'll have to walk solidly for three hours before you've used up the energy in a half pound steak. And most of this

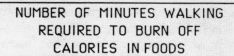

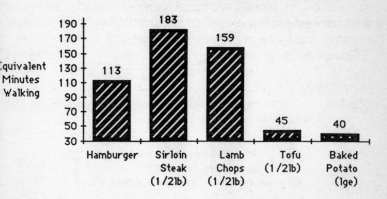

energy, in the form of calories, comes from fat. That's why the fatty foods in the table above will take so long to burn off.

In evolutionary terms, being able to store so much energy in such a highly concentrated form is extremely useful. But for today's lifestyle, it's a big problem. If the body can't use the fat we take in our diet, it will lay it down, just in case it needs it. It never does, of course, because we're busy eating even more fatty foods, and the end result of today's high-fat diet is a high-fat person. With a good chance of an elevated cholesterol level, too.

Certain fats are called *essential* ones, because the body can't manufacture them. They can be found in such foods as wheat germ, most types of seeds, and oils such as safflower, corn and soya. So it would be a good idea to include these items in your diet, while cutting back on other fats.

Just about everyone, even the reluctant food industry, is agreed that we eat too much total fat. But how much is too much? One way of measuring this is to go back to the calorie comparison we've just mentioned. At the moment, we get more than forty per cent of our total energy from the fat in our diet. This is much too high.

Various 'targets' have been suggested by a number of organizations, and the whole area is in danger of becoming confused, which is, no doubt, what some people would like to happen. A sensible goal? At the most, no more than twenty-five per cent to thirty per cent of your total energy should come from fat. But as far as *saturated* fat is concerned, no more than ten per cent of your energy should come from it. That is what the NACNE committee recommended. [12] Even the more conservative COMA [13] committee suggested a maximum of fifteen per cent of energy from saturated fat. In actual weight terms, this is what the COMA report suggested (plotted with shaded lines) and it's compared in this chart with today's *average* intake of fat:

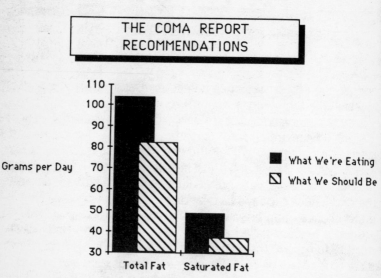

You can see that, even if we were to follow the COMA guidelines, which are extremely cautious, a drastic change would be necessary. But just how easy is it to make this change?

Well, it's going to be very tough. Let's take the upper limit of thirty per cent of calories in our diets coming from all forms of fat. Eating today's popular foods, it's going to be just about impossible for *anyone* to cut their total fat intake back to the suggested level, while at the same time eating a properly balanced diet. This next chart will tell you why.

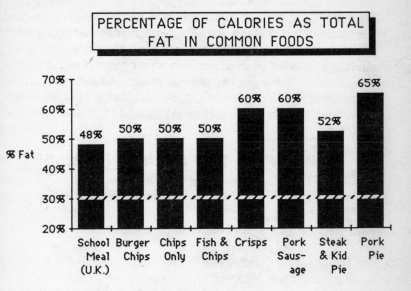

PERCENTAGE OF CALORIES AS TOTAL FAT IN COMMON FOODS

As you can see, there's an awful lot of popular food that has *masses* of fat in it — much more than the thirty per cent that is the recommended top limit, shown on the chart by a shaded line. Do you notice how much of this food is considered to be suitable for children? That's the really chilling part.

All Is Revealed

Now let's try to tie up all these facts about fat we've just considered. All the studies, reports and committees that have had so much publicity in this country recently are basically telling us the same thing — that we've got to cut our *total* fat consumption back from about forty per cent of all calories to about thirty per cent (and you can treat that figure as a maximum).

That's a reduction of twenty-five per cent in our total fat intake. How can we do that?

Although no government committee is going to tell you, the answer is actually devastatingly simple. All you've got to do is cut out meat. Because meat contributes over twenty-five per cent (the government puts it at twenty-seven per cent) of *all* fat in our diet.

Well that was, easy, wasn't it? But of course, there are even more advantages. We've seen the evidence that meat is *very* strongly implicated in coronary heart disease, and that saturated fat (in which meat is naturally rich) is the determining factor in high blood cholesterol, and all the associated dangers.

What Price Your Pound of Flesh?

Even our bumbling, inefficient and perhaps even negligent bureaucrats and government are beginning to admit, today, that the British people are suffering from an epidemic which no-one has ever seen the like of before. In purely financial terms (that's the language our bureaucrats seem to understand the best) it costs our National Health Service well over £215 million each year *just for the drugs* to treat people with coronary heart disease.[14]

And we regularly lose twenty-five million working days *each year* as a result of people being prevented by heart disease from going to work. Other countries, with just as bad a problem, are successfully doing something about it — *why can't we*?

But the true cost of coronary heart disease can't really be measured in terms of mere money. Like hundreds of thousands of other people, I know that from personal experience. For when my father died of a heart attack, after two years spent stubbornly fighting for his life, a whole family died with him. He never had a chance to read the information *you've* just read.

REFERENCES

1. 'Coronary heart Disease in Seven Countries,' Keys, A. (ed) et al, *Circulation*, Supplement 1, Vols XLI and XLII April 1970.
2. 'A Comparison of trends in coronary heart disease mortality in

   Australia, USA and England and Wales', T. Dwyer, B. S. Hetzel,
   International Journal of Epidemiology, Vol 9, no 1.

3. 'Association between dietary changes and mortality rates: Israel 1949
   to 1977 a trend-free regression model', Palgi, A., *American Journal of
   Clinical Nutrition* 34: August 1981, pp. 1569-1583.

4. 'Vegetarianism, dietary fibre and mortality', Michael L. Burr, Peter M.
   Sweetnam, *American Journal of Clinical Nutrition*: 36, pp. 873-877,
   November 1982.

5. 'Dietary intervention study among 30 free-living families in Finland',
   P. Pietinien, R. Doughterty, M. Mutanen, U. Leino, S. Moisio, J. Iacono.
   P. Puska, *Journal of the American Dietetic Association*, March 1984, Vol 84,
   No 3.

6. 'Effect of ingestion of meat on plasma cholesterol of vegetarians', F.
   M. Sacks, A. Donner, W. P. Castelli, J. Gronemeyer, P. Pletka, H. S.
   Margolius, L. Landsberg, E. H. Kass, JAMA, 7 August 1981, Vol 246,
   No 6.

7. 'Effect of cholesterol-lowering diet on mortality from coronary heart
   disease and other causes', O. Turpeinen, *Circulation*, Vol 59 No 1, January
   1979.

8. 'Association between reported diet and all-cause mortality', H. A. Kahn,
   R. L. Phillips, D. A. Snowden, W. Choi, *American Journal of Epidemiology*,
   Vol 119, 5.

9. 'Effect of diet and smoking intervention on the incidence of coronary
   heart disease', I. Hjermann, I. Holme, K. Velve Byre, P. Leren, *The Lancet*,
   Saturday, 12 December 1981.

10. 'Diet, serum cholesterol and death from coronary heart disease', R.
    B. Shekelle, A. M. Shryock, O. Paul, M. Lepper, J. Stamler, S. Liu, W.
    J. Raynor, *New England Journal of Medicine*, 8 January 1981, Vol 304, No 2.

11. 'The Lipid Research Clinics Coronary Primary Prevention Trial Results',
    Lipid Research Clinics Program, JAMA, 20 January1984, Vol 251, No 3.

12. Proposals for nutritional guidelines for health education in Britain,
    NACNE September 1983, Health Education Council.

13. Diet and Cardiovascular Disease, Committee on Medical Aspects of
    Food Policy, HMSO 1984.

14. *Lloyds Bank Review*, October 1982.

6

There's Junk in Your Joint

'You won't quote my name, will you?'

The question came from a vet I was interviewing. Like many other people I have spoken to in the course of researching this book, he was genuinely worried that his livelihood might be threatened if he was seen to speak out publicly against some of our more questionable food production practices. I have found that this self-imposed conspiracy of silence, although subtle, functions very effectively — probably much more so than any Official Secrets Act. Nevertheless, there sometimes comes a point when people can no longer turn a blind eye to what they basically know to be wrong, and this vet was, I thought, ready to speak quite frankly to me. Another vet had suggested that I might profitably talk to him about the black market that I knew existed in antibiotics intended for use on meat animals. After I promised him anonimity, he startled me immediately with an admission he clearly found embarrassing:

'I hardly eat any meat these days, especially not in restaurants. In my opinion, it's not a wholesome product any more, at least much of it isn't. There are too many areas where the consumer is completely at the mercy of the producer, and I don't trust many of the producers or slaughterers I know. They'll do anything they can to make a fast buck, and there's no effective means of policing them. Vets like me are pretty well powerless, the Ministry doesn't have enough money or manpower to enforce the regulations, and most of the legislation doesn't have any teeth in any case.

You wanted to talk to me about food poisoning and antibiotics, well that's a good illustration. We hear a lot about food poisoning cases these days, and in just about every case there's meat or poultry as the root cause. Now who get's the blame when patients in hospital die from it? It's almost always the cook, who's blamed for not cooking the beef long enough or for leaving it out in the open. But that's only partly true, because if the meat wasn't grossly infected with salmonella organisms to start with, there'd be no problem. And an increasing number of virulent strains are becoming more and more resistant to antibiotics. About four out of every five chickens sold in supermarkets are infected with salmonella. I don't see how anyone can really consider that acceptable.

'Do you know how easy it is to cross-infect other food in the kitchen? Well, say the housewife slices into the chicken, and then uses the same knife to slice some bread. She's just spread the infection. Or she puts the chicken down on a work-surface, and then later places some other food on the same spot where the chicken stood. Again, she's transferred the infection. If she pretended to herself that she was handling a lump of raw sewage in a food environment, and took all the necessary precautions, then that would be just about adequate.'

'That's a disgusting thought,' I said. 'But let's get back to antibiotics. Exactly how and why are they used on animals intended for human consumption?'

'Alright,' he answered. 'There are three categories of use, but the distinctions are frequently blurred. First, there's therapeutic use. That means if a cow gets sick, just like a human, I'll give her something to clear it up. Second, there's prophylactic, which means that in the case I've just mentioned I'd probably give the rest of the herd something to prevent *them* from catching it, too. And third, there's the use of antibiotics for growth promotion. It gets mixed in their feed, and they're taking it in all the time, whether or not they're sick. I don't usually get involved in that.'

'Why not?' I asked. 'Don't you control the drugs that the animals in your care receive, rather like a doctor does for humans?'

He gave a sardonic smile. 'It's not the same thing at all. For one thing, there's no applicable law.'

'But surely,' I objected, 'there must be some legal control over the antibiotics that animals are allowed to receive?'

'There are no effective regulations,' he said. 'That's the problem. There's no control, and no practical monitoring whatsoever. Bascially, antibiotics are divided into two classes — those that the farmer can give to his animals himself, without asking me, and those that need my authority. Let's take the first group. Lincomycin, spiramycin, tylosin, virginiamycin — and several others — are freely available, over the counter, and already mixed into animal feeds. The calf rearer can buy them without even mentioning it to me. Something like lincomycin, for example, is a 'last resort' drug for use on humans, when there's resistance to penicillin. But a farmer can go right out and use as much of the stuff as he wants to, and damn the consequences.'

'What *are* the consequences?' I asked.

'In a word,' he said, 'resistance. There's intrinsic resistance, when prolonged exposure to sub-clinical doses of an antibiotic produces organisms that are now resistant to it. Now, when these organisms with newly-acquired resistance infect humans, the doctors can't use the old antibiotic to treat them. It just doesn't work any more. That's one problem, but there's another called "cross-resistance", which is potentially even worse. That happens when one organism passes on its own resistance to a certain drug to a new organism. So the old antibiotic is now useless against two or more organisms, not just one. Because of these two problems, doctors are taught to give short, sharp antibiotic treatment to humans, and not to spread it out over long periods as a prophylactic dose, except under very special circumstances. But no-one controls the way antibiotics are used on the farm. That's why we talk of a "reservoir" of resistance. We know there's a large reservoir of E. Coli in calves and pigs that are very resistant to most antibiotics, and we know that resistance can be "donated" by them to more dangerous organisms, such as salmonellae. But no-one's responsible for trying to eliminate this cross-resistance.'

'But you are, aren't you?' I asked him. 'As a vet, it's your responsibility to, isn't it?'

'Oh yes, it probably is in theory,' he said. 'But there's a great deal of difference between theory and practice. I'm in business. I'm not going to turn my customers away, you know. If they don't get what they want from me, they'll get it somewhere else, and they're not slow to threaten me. There was a case just recently. Some feedstuff representatives were calling on calf rearers in this area trying to sell a milk-replacement that had been medicated with one particular antibiotic that is practically the only weapon we have against a notoriously resistant strain of salmonella that's very common just at the moment. If this strain — for your information, it's called PT 204c — acquires resistance to nitrofuran, which is the antibiotic, then we're really in trouble. The feedstuff reps are fools who ought to know better. But what can I do? It's an impossible situation. That's what happened to the tetracyclines. They were a powerful, broad-spectrum range of antibiotics that were very widely used in human medicine. But now, there are so many resistant strains, they're not nearly so useful. But the farmers keep on using them, and the vets keep on prescribing them, because they're being commercially pressured to do so.'

'Apart from food poisoning with salmonella,' I asked, 'what other organisms can acquire this type of resistance?'

He shrugged. 'There's really no limit. Gonorrhoea, meningitis, enteric fever, enteritis, organisms that cause septicaemia in the blood stream, abscesses in the lungs, liver or bones, even the heart — just a small selection.'

'But has it actually been proven that this can happen?' I asked.

'Scientifically there's no doubt whatsoever. Take a look at this.' He went to a bookshelf, pulled out some bound magazines and indicated an article.

'It's not easy to undertake studies like this, because they're expensive, and take a lot of manpower. But this one took place in the States a couple of years ago, and I doubt very much whether the situation would be any better in Britain.'

I looked at the report. It was produced by the Centre for Disease Control, in Georgia, famous for its pioneering detective work.[1] These are some of the points they made:

● About twenty-five per cent of human salmonella infections are now resistant to drug therapy. This isn't confined to just one drug, they're *multiple* resistant. This percentage is steadily increasing all the time.

● Astonishingly, half the antibiotics now commercially produced are fed to food animals, largely for 'disease prevention' or 'growth promotion.'

● They tracked 312 people who were infected with drug-resistant salmonella. Subsequently, thirteen of them died from it. This is a mortality rate of four per cent — *twenty-one* times higher than the death-rate from old-fashioned, non-resistant salmonella.

● They tracked one outbreak of salmonella poisoning in Minneapolis, and found that the factor that all the patients had in common was that they had eaten hamburger from a herd of cattle that had been given "sub-therapeutic" doses of chlortetracycline. The "trigger" that precipitated the outbreak was when each patient took a penicillin-derived drug. Then, in a way that still isn't completely understood, something happened to upset the delicate internal balance of micro-organisms in their bodies. Suddenly, the drug-resistant salmonella was dormant no longer, and rapidly flared up to cause a massive infection. Out of ten cases, one person died.

● They concluded the study by stating that 'antimicrobial-resistant organisms of animal origin cause serious human illness. We emphasise the need for more prudent used of antimicrobials in humans and animals.'

'What's the picture in Britain?', I asked.

'No different. The drug companies, and other financially-interested organisations, employ vets like me to provide prescriptions to farmers, and they do what they're told to do. We know that salmonella resistance is growing. Have you heard of typhoid fever? Well, that's caused by a strain of salmonella. It's treated with chloramphenicol, but over ten per cent of salmonella organisms are now resistant to it. The whole thing just goes round and round.

Because animal excrement is now processed to make feedstuff for other animals, we're just reinfecting more and more animals all the time. Chickens are now being fed their own excrement to about fifty per cent of their total intake of food, it's very economical. But it means that contaminants, such as drugs, hormones, pesticides and antibiotics are getting more and more concentrated each time they go through. And we know that anything between a quarter and a half of all feedstuff is contaminated. But what can we do about it?'

'Well,' I said, 'I suppose that's *your* problem. Can you give me any information about other potential hazards in this sort of drug misuse?'

'Resistance is the problem that's had most publicity. And there's no doubt that it's extremely serious. In the past six years, the number of reported cases of salmonella poisoning has doubled, to about 20,000 a year. But that's just the tip of the iceberg, because salmonella doesn't usually get diagnosed, sometimes it can be as mild as sickness and diarrhoea.

'There could be two other problems with antibiotics. First, there could be a direct toxic effect. Do you know what a "casualty" animal is? Well, its one that's sent to the slaughterhouse, although it really shouldn't go. It may have almost any disease. So the farmer doses it up with a strong antibiotic to keep it on its feet for the next few hours until it's slaughtered, and you've got a piece of meat that's pretty well medicated, particularly if you happen to get the part of its body that received the injection on your plate. If you're unlucky, the toxic effect might include blurring of vision, lung disorders, renal failure, or just depression. But it might not even stop there, because a woman could pass it on to her child in her milk.

'The second human problem is a hypersensitivity reaction. Antibiotics that are added to foodstuffs as "disease preventatives" or simply as "growth promoters" are, of course, at sub-therapeutic doses, and over a long period of time. But we know from human studies that side-effects are more related to length of exposure rather than to high dosage. If a patient is receiving an antibiotic over a long period, they have to be closely monitored, because reactions are notoriously unpredictable, and their onset can be very sudden indeed. The symptoms can include widespread lesions of the skin, and fatal hepatitis. But who'd think of associating these symptoms with meat consumption?'

'It seems like a treadmill we can't get off,' I said. 'What do you think will happen?'

'You're right,' he agreed. 'It's a vicious circle, but we've gone too far now to turn back. You see, once vets were people who looked after the well-being of animals, both farm and domestic. But now, we just supress the disease until it's time for the animal to be killed. That's all the farmer requires of us. Our antibiotics and other drugs kill off the good organisms, as well as the bad. So a calf, for example, doesn't have a chance to acquire natural immunity from her mother, as wild animals do. The beneficial intestinal bacteria just can't grow, and it means that our antibiotics are actually making that calf more vulnerable to disease, not less. But we can't stop now. Think what an epidemic we'd have if we did. It means, of course, that the animals that go to make your daily meat aren't necessarily *healthy* animals — they just don't have clinical signs of disease. There's a big difference.'

'What about illegal supplies of these drugs?' I asked.

He smiled. 'You wouldn't really think it was necessary, would you? After all, a farmer can get just about anything he wants now, in any case. But there'll always be a black market, especially if it's cheaper. And if they ever get round to banning any of these drugs, then that's sure to stimulate under the counter trade. I don't think you'll ever get rid of it.'

I could see from his expression that I wasn't going to get any further with this line of questioning. It was the usual reaction I had had from just about everyone I mentioned the subject to. Everyone knew it went on, but no-one would point the finger. And in a way, I agreed with him. The black market, even though it provided possibly dangerous drugs in impure form or high concentrations, didn't really seem so bad when compared to the state of affairs that exists quite legally. The whole thing seemed to be an enormous black market, with little practical control and a tremendous potential for abuse. I asked one final question.

'Are there any other drugs that are commonly used and might have the same implications for public health?'

'Where do you want to begin?' he answered. 'There's DDT, for one.'

'But I'm sure that's banned, isn't it?' I said, surprised.

'Not for sheep dips,' he replied. 'In fact it's compulsory, twice a year. There's little doubt that the DDT derivatives, such as Lindane, for example, persist in the meat. And they accumulate in your body. If the sheep is going for export, the producer has to sign a certificate saying that they haven't been dipped in the preceding six weeks. That's all that's required.'

'But isn't there any inspection?' I asked.

'There are two sorts of slaugherhouses', he told me. 'Ones that kill for the export market, and ones that kill for the home market. The export ones have to be of a much higher standard. Samples of the meat are analysed for hormones, antibiotics, and other drug residues. Even so, only a small amount of the meat is sampled. But for the home market, the standards are not so strict. For one thing, the inspectors just don't have the time or money. An inspector may only visit a slaughterhouse once a week, and providing things are alright when he calls, there won't be any problems. So it's really up to the farmers and the slaughtermen to be good boys. Of course — ' he added with a knowing look, 'they always are.'

At that point, we finished talking. The conversation was quite typical of many that I'd had with people working inside the meat industry — on the one hand, concern about the many scandals and abuses taking place right under their noses; and on the other hand, a feeling of powerlessness to do anything about the situation. Subsequently, further conversations with more people working inside the industry have revealed even more causes for concern. A few of them follow.

The Allergy Connection

It is known that, at *extremely* small doses, antibiotics can provoke quite severe allergic reactions in some people. One case, for example, of dermatitis due to hypersensitivity to penicillin has been reported in a person after ingesting only 0.03 unit per millilitre of milk containing slight penicillin residue.[2] We know that cases of allergy — including asthma and eczema — have increased alarmingly over the past few decades, roughly in line with increased antibiotic use.

Among children, especially, the situation is definitely much worse than it used to be. Asthma is *three times* more common today amongst children than it was when their parents were young. And eczema is *six times* more common. Whilst the precipitating factors are likely to be complex, it is quite possible that the "background medication" they receive through meat and milk could well have something to do with it.

The Scale of the Problem

It is very difficult to accurately assess the amount of residue present in meat offered for sale in this country (or, particularly, in processed meat products). The tiny amount of sampling that is carried out in slaughterhouses really doesn't allow accurate statistical analysis to be done (except, of course, in slaughterhouses licensed for export — there the standards are much stricter). But one recent inquiry showed that anything from twenty-six per cent to fifty-eight per cent of pork meat contained detectable antibiotic residue. The liver and other organs were found to be consistently higher in residues than any other area. Thus, "offal" meat, which was once considered to be nutritionally good and cheap to purchase, should be regarded with suspicion, because it is in these organs that residues will tend to accumulate. Of course, offal (including brains, rectum, eyes, lips, testes, ovaries, feet, lungs, etc) are usually processed into "meat products", and so it is no longer easy to avoid these parts of the animal's body.

Cancer Rears its Head — Again

Some anti-microbial agents (not necessarily antibiotics, but used in much the same way to treat infection) also have the capacity to cause cancer or mutations. This has been experimentally proven on laboratory animals. So what is the 'safe' dose that humans may receive? The answer is that there is no safe dose. As an American research paper on this subject says:

> Until the opposite is proven, it must be assumed that any chemical that gives rise to tumours in experimental animals would also do so in humans (International Agency for Research on Cancer, 1983). Another generally accepted postulate is that for a given carcinogen there is no dose so low as to be considered safe. In other words, any amount of a carcinogen, however minute, would lead to tumour development in some individuals in a sufficiently large population after a sufficiently long latency period. [3]

So *some* people will develop cancerous tumours. The only question that the authorities have to answer is, is the number of people likely to develop tumours sufficiently low to justify the risk? Of course, that is a very cynical viewpoint. You may consider that *any* risk is too much, particularly when you bear in mind that *we're* taking the risk so that the meat industry can swell their own profits by stimulating unnaturally fast weight gain on their animals.

The Bottom Line

The whole question of antibiotics is not, fundamentally, about animal health. It's about high turnover, fast re-stocking times, rapid weight gain, disease suppression, and all the other factors that are so important to today's technological meat machine. Antibiotics are just one more tool that helps the industry to maximize its profit margins. The farm vet is no longer a professional person, with an independent code of ethics — he's been roped into the business too, either as a 'consultant' to a pharmaceutical company, or by forced coercion from his major customers. He has become a technologist, whose only task is to keep animals free from the symptoms of disease (note — I did not say healthy) until they can be profitably slaughtered. More and more vets are feeling unhappy about their new role, but there's not much they can really do about it if they want to earn their wages. As always, the consumer's real interests are right at the bottom of the pile. There's only one way they benefit, in fact — and that's by having an artificially low price tag on the meat they buy. For there's no doubt about it — if meat were to be produced in an ethical way (possibly a contradiction in terms) it would cost many times more.

But what is the *real* price we're paying? If we're saving a few pounds at the supermarket checkout, and paying for it with our health (or that of our children), that — surely — is a terrible price, and simply too much for us to afford.

REFERENCES

1. 'Drug-resistant salmonella from animals fed antimicrobials', S. D. Holmberg, M. T. Osterholm, K. A. Senger, M. L. Cohen, *New England Journal of Medicine*, Vol 311 no 10, 6 September, 1984.
2. A Bookshelf on Veterinary Public Health, AJPH, April 1973, Vol 63, no 4.
3. Survey of Animal Drugs with carcinogenic properties, A. Somogyi, *Food Additives and Contaminants*, 1984, Vol 1, no 2, pp 81-87.

7

How Not to Wreck a Marriage

As we sat down at the table for lunch, I was aware of a very tense atmosphere. I'd known my friends Michael and Kate for two or three years, and I'd always thought they were happily married — but now, the feeling was definitely icy.

Kate was a good cook, and she'd prepared a truly mouth-watering meal that included some of my favourite food — hummus and pita bread as a starter, a huge bowl of green salad with Kate's special dressing, and I could smell a magnificent curry gently simmering in the kitchen. It looked as if we were in for a good meal. But then I glanced over to Michael, and it seemed to me that maybe he didn't quite share my enthusiasm. Kate picked up my thoughts.

'Mike wants his meat,' she said, and her voice was quite sharp. 'I've told him I'm not going to cook it for him any more. I don't have time to cook two lots of meals, and I don't see why he can't eat like the rest of us.'

'Oh,' I said. I didn't particularly want to get involved in a dispute between husband and wife. But I also didn't want to have a perfectly good meal ruined by a bad atmosphere. Plucking up my courage, I said to Mike; 'D'you miss it that badly, Mike?'

For a moment, I thought he wasn't going to answer. Then, with a visible effort, he began to tell me about it. 'Kate hasn't eaten meat for six months now, but she's always cooked it for me when I've asked her. Now she's gone on strike. I know this is supposed to be a healthier way of eating, but I don't see why I should literally have it rammed down my throat. I just like the taste of meat, that's all. I guess I'll have to eat out from now on.'

Mike was clearly feeling sorry for himself, and there wasn't much I could do to change things. It didn't seem as if he was in the mood to discuss it. But towards the end of the meal, after Mike had twiddled with a few lettuce leaves, and left most of his food on his plate, I decided to have another go.

'Look, what's wrong with you?' I said. 'You've left most of your food, and you're not going to tell me that it didn't taste good, because I won't believe you. So why don't you get it off your chest?'

He gave a wry grin. 'Maybe I *was* acting bit childish. You're right, there's nothing wrong with the food, its okay. But I just miss the meat. You know I work hard, and feel I've got to eat something substantial, or I won't have enough energy to carry me through the day. I need the protein.'

'But you *know* there's lots of protein in what we just ate,' I objected. He was also confusing his protein with his energy requirements, but I wasn't about to give him a lecture in home economics.

'I suppose there is,' he agreed. 'But I'm used to meat, and I can't do without it. I guess I'm hooked!'

Kate gave me a despairing glance, and went out into the kitchen. Mike's tone of voice became serious.

'Look,' he said. 'This happens at just about every meal now. I'm not eating properly, and I'm fed up with it. One of us is going to have to give way, and it's not going to be me. Things have never been so bad between Kate and me. I'm beginning to wonder if we're really compatible.'

I'm afraid this story — which is a true one — didn't have a happy ending. A few weeks afterwards Kate moved out, and I doubt whether they'll ever get back together. And I know that other people have had similar problems in this situation. So — to try to prevent it happening to *you* — here are some ideas that other couples have successfully used to get over the 'meat barrier'.

Do It Together

If one of you is contemplating doing away with meat in your diet, the most important thing is to talk it through, together, before you actually change anything. Don't underestimate the impact this change will have on your lifestyles. Eating is one of the most fundamental of all human activities, and any major change is bound to have considerable repercussions. By talking it through together, and planning it together, you'll ensure that all the consequences of your choice are good ones.

I've found from personal experience that the couples who seem to have most problems at this time are the ones who *don't* normally share other things together — where the wife always does the cooking, for example, and the husband always does the eating. Conversely, the couples I know who share the food preparation are invariably the ones who get the most pleasure out of it — and there's at least as much pleasure in making food as in eating it. It's easy to forget that, with so much instant and fast food around these days. So try rediscovering this special sort of togetherness for yourselves. If that sounds like a tall order, have a go at some of the suggestions that follow.

A useful trick to involve males in the kitchen (who may have been badly spoiled by their mothers) is to appeal to their vanity. Certain aspects of cookery are more 'technical' than others, and these can be presented as an intellectual challenge for them. Here are some ideas:

● Give him a book about making soya milk and tofu (soya bean curd) and ask him to ''explain'' it to you. This is a fascinating process, and will provide him with many happy hours! Hopefully, it'll also produce some food too!

● Certain recipes have a macho sound to them, so ask him to try them out for you. In the same way as men enjoy grilling and barbecuing things, get him to try all the many different forms of curry (there are thousands), barbecue foods, bread (it's very physical), anything with alcohol in, etc.

● Tell him that he should think about opening a restaurant. Most men have their own distinct ideas about this, and you never know, he might just end up doing it! Even if he doesn't, he'll have learnt something useful in the kitchen.

● Try creating recipes together. You can start by asking him to suggest 'improvements' to standard recipes, and then ask him to show you what he means. It'll set you both thinking!

● When you're feeling reasonably confident, throw a small party at which he can show off his newly acquired skills.

Does it take longer to prepare? That's a question that gets asked a lot. In the early days, of course, it's bound to take longer, because you'll be experimenting with new recipes and doing a lot of learning. However, there are very many meat-free dishes that take less than ten minutes from start to finish, and you'll find these useful when you're pushed for time. Also, remember that you can use your freezer to keep left-overs, which again can be used at short notice. Personally, I don't mind if I'm working in the kitchen for half an hour or so — it's more interesting than being stuck in front of the television.

Know Why You're Doing It

You will be quite amazed at the amount of interest your decision to go meat-free will create amongst your friends (and it'll probably make you a lot of new ones). It's certainly a fashionable thing to do at the moment, which may, of course, put some people off. You might even get fed up with people asking you about it. Other people are bound to be extremely curious, and many of them may even give it a try too, as a direct result of talking to you. The first question that you're inevitably bound to get asked is:

'Why don't you eat meat any more?'

It always helps to have a ready answer (there are enough of them in this book!). Since this is a matter of personal preference, you'll just have to sort this one out between yourselves. Out of interest, I'll tell you what I usually say:

'Mainly because it's healthier, because I don't need to kill other creatures in order to eat, because it wastes a lot less of the world's resources, and because I'm just crazy about ratatouille.'

I usually find that covers pretty much everything! After a few seconds, when my questioner has fully recovered, they'll probably pick one of those subjects, and want to talk more about it. That's fine with me, it's a good way of getting to know people.

What Shall We Tell the Children?

This is not always so easy. Children can be extremely conservative in their tastes, and sometimes nothing will change them. But, like Joe, who you've already met, many children *are* deciding to reject meat these days, and you may find that, after discussing it with them, you've got an unexpected ally.

Their age is perhaps the most important factor. Leaving aside the nutritional aspects, which we'll consider later, most young children (up to seven or eight) won't cause any problems, and will thrive on a fresh food diet, tending towards the bland.

But after that age the problems may start. Children today come under such intensive pressure, from advertising and from their peer groups, that any non-conformity may be almost impossible for them to sustain. You can't expect kids of this age to be unduly concerned about their own health (although *you* should be, because you're setting up a lifetime's eating habits for them). Nor can they easily grasp the economic arguments of the gross waste of world resources, although they'll be quick to empathize with pictures of famine and starvation.

The only answer here is to tell them the truth — about where their hamburger comes from. I remember being genuinely shocked when I was a child after learning that meat was literally 'dead animals'. Somehow, I though that meat was co-operatively produced between humans and animals, with no violence and no slaughter. Perhaps that idea wasn't really so stupid, because we *do* give children that impression. Those jolly, smiling, half-human, half-animal caricatures of piglets that you see decorating butchers' shops, and the happy pig wearing a straw boater and striped butcher's apron gaily wielding an axe — all these images are pure marketing fantasy, intended to conceal the ugly truth of the slaughterhouse from us.

The vast majority of children feel a naturally close kinship with animals, which can be greatly enhanced if they keep pets. Unlike adults, kids can be totally unhypocritical. If you are honest enough to tell them the truth about the process of meat production, then you are putting them in a situation where they can take a properly informed decision for themselves. They will quickly work out for themselves that a tremendous contradiction exists between the 'cuddly' image of animals that the meat industry 'sells' them on the one hand, and the harsh reality of meat production that exists on the other. But we *must* have the courage to be absolutely honest with them. It's far too easy just to let them carry on living in the fantasy world that's been created for them, where animals are cuddly friends and where 'meat' is a disembodied object that comes nicely pre-packaged from the freezer shelf in the supermarket. That isn't being honest, it's just conning them.

So what do you tell them? Again, it depends on their age. It's probably a good idea to find out how *they* think meat is produced first, and then correct any inaccuracies they may have. That, by itself, may be enough to get them thinking for themselves — which is often all you need to do. The moral justification, if they are interested, is quite simple. They wouldn't kill and eat a cow or a chicken for themselves, would they? So it's not right to pay *other* people to kill animals, just because you're not prepared to do it yourself. You could also point out that adults frequently try to avoid the consequences of their own decisions in this highly irrational way — there are plenty more examples.

Eating with Friends

If you're invited for a meal at a friend's house, it's probably best to warn them in advance that your food preferences have changed, and so avoid any problems. Otherwise, you might find yourself stuck in a situation that I've sometimes seen people in — being forced to make do with a parsley and lettuce leaf garnish all evening ('It's alright, I'm not really hungry'). Or, even worse, being so embarrassed for your host/hostess that you miserably swallow the meat course in painful silence. You can avoid both of these difficult situations by checking in advance — once is all it takes, and they'll know in future. There are a number of options open to you, usually a phone call something like this is all that is necessary: 'By the way, I thought I'd give you a call just to let you know in advance that I've[we've] given up eating meat. I hope it won't be too difficult for you?' Usually, your friend will thank you for being so thoughtful and letting them know. Just occasionally, they will be stumped for an answer, in which case you have various possibilities. You could offer to drop by beforehand for a chat with a few recipe books, which could be another enjoyable social occasion in its own right. Of, if you're feeling brave, you could offer to cook something yourself, and bring it for everyone to try (be warned — cook enough, or you won't get any yourself!). Whatever you and your friend decide, it's likely to be the conversational and culinary centrepiece of the evening, and will almost certainly make you the party's expert, who everyone will want to talk to!

Eating Out

According to the latest information, over 25 per cent of all restaurants in the United Kingdom now have at least one meat-free main course meal on their menu. The picture is getting better and better all the time, so you shouldn't have too much difficulty when it comes to eating out.

Most restaurateurs know a good thing when they see one, and a meatless meal is actually more profitable for them to prepare and serve than all the fuss and wastage involved in cooking meat. So more and more restaurants are quickly realizing that what's good for their customers is also good for their bank account. Most Indian, Chinese, Italian, Mexican, Greek, Jewish, Middle Eastern and of course health food restaurants will prove particularly easy to eat in. If you don't see anything you fancy on the menu ('Oh no! Not *another* cheese salad!') get to see the owner or the head chef, who in my experience will be only too delighted to try and expand his culinary repertoire. You may even get to try some unique ethnic dish that is usually reserved for 'the regulars' (that's how I first got to try tofu in a Chinese restaurant).

Don't let overbearing restaurant staff make you feel uncomfortable. It's extremely rude for them to say (as they used to in the past, but almost never do now): 'Why didn't you telephone before you came? We might have been able to do something for you.'

This is a calculated attempt to make you feel like a social leper, who ought to warn people in advance of his likely movements so that others can take avoiding action. Whenever this happened to me, I told them that if they knew anything at all about cooking (which they clearly don't) they'd know that it takes *less*, not more time to prepare. And you could try asking them what they *would* have prepared for you if you'd have phoned. I bet you'd get the following answer:

YOU: 'What can you do for me without meat?'
WAITER: 'Anything you want. What would you like?'
YOU: 'Well I don't know what you can do, what do you suggest?'
WAITER: 'We can do anything. What do you want?'

And so it goes on. This sort of conversation is infuriating and unfortunately is a sign that you've found a really poor restaurant. What it means is that the waiter can't be bothered to go and speak to the chef, and see what he suggests. So he's trying to intimidate you to having the easy option — the inevitable cheese salad or omelette — which is precisely what you *don't* want when you're eating out. And even if you *do* come up with the name of a dish you fancy, nine times out of ten he'll tell you that it can't be made. The answer is to call for the chef or the owner — or (my personal preference) *walk out*!

I have no hesitation whatsoever in walking out of a restaurant, and neither should you. There are plenty more to choose from, and if no-one has taken any trouble over your food or your service, then you have a duty to show the management that their standards are slipping. Similarly, don't hesitate to send food back that's indifferent — you're paying enough for it, and you'll find you get amazingly better service next time!

However, that really is the ultimate deterrent. Most of the time you'll find that eating out has regained a fresh novelty for you and you'll discover a whole new cuisine — you may get some stimulating ideas for cooking at home, too. And, because you're not just run-of-the-mill customers, you'll find that the staff take much more interest in you, and the chef will also take more personal pride in making you something, and he'll want to know whether or not you liked it (remember to tell him!) I've often been with a mixed meat/non-meat party where everyone has enviously agreed that my food has seemed much better and more attractively presented than other people's. That's the reason why.

Be Prepared for the Nuts!

I believe in being assertive when it comes to personal matters such as food. I *don't* believe that anyone (such as a restaurant, an acquaintance, or even an entire food industry) has the right to tell you what to do. Unfortunately, at some stage you're almost bound to come up against some ill-inspired personal criticism, perhaps from family or just casual acquaintances, so let's consider various ways of handling it.

The first thing to realize is that there's always a reason for any criticism that's sent in your direction. If you can discover what it is, you're half-way to overcoming it. I've been at perfectly normal parties when suddenly someone will make a terrifically aggressive and provocative remark that's obviously intended to hurt those of us who didn't happen to be devouring a lump of animal flesh at that moment. Why do people behave like that?

Perhaps you've already come up against that sort of person. They may sneer at you if you're wearing leather shoes, or tell you that carrots scream when they're boiled, or make some other mocking remark. Personally, I believe we're dealing here with the phenomenon psychologists call 'projected guilt'. The classic example that psychologists tell each other about the lady who, when shown a series of random ink blots, exclaims to the psychologist: 'How dare you, sir! How dare you show such disgusting pictures to me!'

The fault lies mainly in the eye of the beholder, and perhaps you should point that out if it ever happens to you.

On the whole, it's probably best not to be provoked, if you can help it. After all, why should anyone get their perverse entertainment at your expense? There are actually several good ways of handling this sort of situation. The first is to treat the question absolutely seriously (with more seriousness than it really deserves), explore the reasons that lie behind it, and give it a precise answer. That will impress anyone else who happens to be listening, and may win you some grudging admiration from your assailant. Another way is to simply put the questioner down by poking some fun at them. Of course, they'll hate you even more if you do this!

My personal preference is to treat any critical remarks as veiled requests for information, until, of course, it's quite obvious that the questioner is lusting after your blood, when you'll have to do something to defend yourself. If you're prepared to ignore any preliminary insults (that some people, possibly insecure ones, feel they've got to make almost as a formality), then you may well strike up quite a good conversation. This dialogue took place when I was a guest at a wedding, and is a good example:

QUESTIONER: 'I see you're not eating any meat'.

ME (examining plate): 'Goodness me, you're quite right, I'm not'.

QUESTIONER: 'Is that for religious reasons?'

ME:' No. Are you *eating* meat for religious reasons, then?'

QUESTIONER: 'No, I just like it. Why aren't you eating what the rest of us are eating?'

ME: 'There are several other people eating the same as me. I hope it doesn't make you feel too uncomfortable'.

QUESTIONER: 'They say that carrots scream, you know, when you boil them'.

ME: 'Well, personally, I tend to eat them raw. But I doubt whether they scream. They don't have a central nervous system, so they don't have the same ability to suffer that animals and humans do. But a lot of people are cutting down on their meat these days, often for health reasons. How about you?'

QUESTIONER: 'Well, I suppose I *am* eating less than I used to.

It doesn't seem to taste the same as it used to. But I wouldn't know what to replace it with.'

And so we got into a discussion of meat 'replacements', and I told him about some of my favourite dishes, and we struck up a good conversation that several other people joined in with. By standing your ground quite firmly, but not responding to an aggressive preliminary, you stand the best chance of avoiding a clash *and* maybe making a friend. Go out and make it work for you!

8

The Deadly Duo: Diabetes and Hypertension

Quiet Killer No. 1: Diabetes

The Risk

Today's children are *six* times more likely to contract diabetes than their parents were. Because diabetes is no longer the killer that it once was, we tend to overlook it as a serious disease. But it *is* serious, because it is often a factor in the development of premature coronary disease, kidney failure, or blindness. Just because we have learnt to control it's symptoms (through insulin injections), we seem to think that it's no longer a major public health problem, which it most certainly still is.

What is Diabetes?

Diabetes mellitus is a metabolic disease in which there is a relative insulin deficiency resulting in the faulty metabolism of carbohydrate. In particular, the body finds it difficult or impossible to convert blood sugar (glucose) into usable energy, leading to an accumulation of sugar in the blood, spilling over into the urine. This is why the words 'diabetes mellitus' literally mean 'sweet leaking'.

The body normally produces the hormone insulin to undertake this metabolism, but in a diabetic person insulin production may be insufficient.

Before the discovery of insulin, diabetes was considered to be invariably fatal, and most patients died within a short time of its diagnosis. Diabetes can be treated effectively today, although it does increase the risk of suffering other serious illnesses, such as cardiovascular disease, eye disorders, gangrene and other circulatory problems, nerve and muscle problems, and an increased susceptibility to ordinary infections. Some authorities believe that diabetes-related complications are the third largest cause of death today.

One of the symptoms of the onset of diabetes is the frequent urge to urinate. Other symptoms include continuous thirst; drinking large volumes of liquids; hunger and weight loss; weakness and fatigue; itches; loose teeth; depressed sex drive; skin disorders; blurring of vision; a degeneration of the functions of the eyes, kidneys, circulation and nervous systems.

Those at Risk

It has been established that a susceptibility to diabetes can be hereditary, and obesity is strongly implicated in its development. Almost half of all adult diabetics are overweight. In Japan, almost all Sumo wrestlers become diabetic before they are thirty-five years old, and it is strongly suspected that this is induced by the amazingly high-fat diet they are given. Women are more likely to become diabetic than men, particularly between the ages of forty-five and seventy, although diabetes in men is usually a more serious condition. Non-whites are also more at risk.

The Evidence

Traditionally, it was supposed that diabetics should reduce their carbohydrate consumption (sugars, plant foods) and increase their protein and fat consumption (dairy food, meat). However, in view of the connection between diabetes and cardiovascular disease, this treatment came under increasing attack, as diabetics are particularly vulnerable to high blood fat levels. It therefore seems to make more sense to restrict total fat intake, whilst reducing *simple* carbohydrates and boosting *complex* carbohydrates.

Research at Oxford confirms this. The aim was to see if what you ate had anything to do with the 'peaks and troughs' in your blood sugar level. Two groups were compared before eating, and found to have an average of 160mg of blood sugar per 100ml of blood. One group was fed a low fibre meal, low in complex carbohydrates — quite typical of the 'junk' food that many people eat today. Their blood sugar level more than doubled very quickly, rising sharply to 380mg, and staying above the 300mg level for more than two hours.

The other group was given a high fibre meal, high in complex carbohydrates — such as are found in vegetables, pulses and cereals. There was a distinctly slow rise in blood sugar to 260mg, and then a slow return to the original level. The complex fibres in the second group's diet had slowed down and smoothed out the body's absorption of carbohydrates, thus avoiding a sudden rush of insulin to deal with a high sugar level.

In addition, some fibres — such as oat bran, and various beans such as kidney, pinto and haricot — seem to be able to lower blood cholesterol levels, which could help a diabetic to reduce the cardiovascular risk. Since animal proteins contain large amounts of fat, it therefore seems possible that a low-meat, high-vegetable diet would be of benefit to some patients.

Existing Diabetics Benefit from High Fibre

Further evidence comes from a study carried out at the Veterans Administration medical Centre in Lexington.[1] Two diets were compared for the treatment of non-obese diabetic men, all of whom required insulin therapy. The 'control' diet provided twenty grams per day of plant fibre — an average Western diet. The other diet included over three times as much fibre — sixty-five grams a day, and was also high in carbohydrates. The researchers found that the men on high fibre, high carbohydrate diets needed seventy-three per cent *less* insulin therapy than those on ordinary diets — quite an amazing reduction. They also found that the average blood pressures of those on high fibre diets were ten per cent lower than those on ordinary diets.

Can a Meat-Free Diet Help to Prevent Diabetes?

What can you do to try and prevent the disease in the first place? Recent research has produced some exciting new evidence. [2] The School of Public Health at the University of Minnesota started a massive study of the subject in 1960, which lasted for twenty-one years and involved 25,698 adult Americans. They belonged to the Seventh-day Adventist church, a group of people we've already encountered as being well-known for their low meat consumption (fifty per cent of them never eat it).

The findings of this study showed that people on meat-free diets has a *substantially* reduced risk (forty-five per cent) of contracting diabetes compared to the population as a whole.

They found that people who consumed meat ran over *twice* the risk of dying from a diabetes-related cause. The correlation between meat consumption and diabetes was found to be particularly strong in males. The study was carefully designed to eliminate confusion arising from confounding factors, such as over- or under-weight,

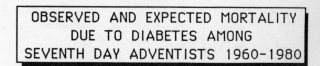

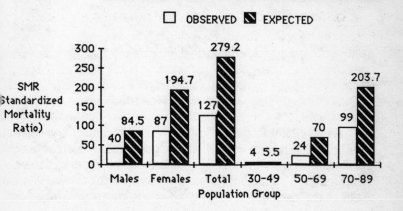

other dietary habits, or amount of physical activity. By comparing deaths from diabetes among Adventists to deaths in the same age- and sex-specific groups in the general U.S. population, it was possible to compare what *actually* happened to what *should* have happened if the Adventists died in the same way as the whole population. See the way it charts out on page 129.

You can see that there is, of course, a striking difference between the number of people who were *expected* to die (heavy shading) and the number of people who *actually* died (light shading). But the study went even further than this. By analysing death-certificates over the period under study, it was possible to assess the *increased risk* of dying from a diabetic illness that those who consumed meat ran. This is how it looks graphically:

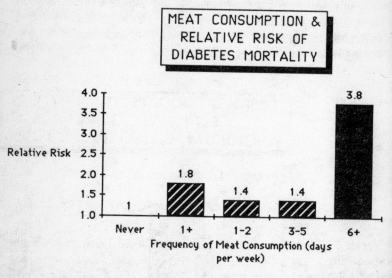

This shows that taking *any* meat in the diet increases the risk, on average, by 1.8 times. For 'light' meat eaters, people who only eat meat once to twice per week, the relative risk compared to a non-meat user is 1.4 times. But for *heavy* users — six or more times a week — the risk rises steeply to 3.8 times. It looks like a bad bet.

The Verdict

It seems that those who suffer from diabetes might well investigate the beneficial possibilities of a largely meat-free diet. For those who wish to reduce their susceptibility to the disease, evidence suggests that a meat-free diet could help considerably.

Quiet Killer No. 2: Hypertension

Hypertension is the medical name for high blood-pressure. Like diabetes, medicine has made impressive progress in the clinical treatment of hypertension, and this has resulted in a decline in mortality from strokes, for example, over the last three decades. But that's not the full picture. A recent survey among 3,000 Scots in the forty-five to sixty-four age group revealed that nearly forty per cent of them had high blood-pressure. And we know that raised blood-pressure is one of the key risk factors in the development of heart disease and cerebrovascular disease. The United Kingdom government estimate that over 240,000 people die every year as a result of a hypertension-related disease. [3] Put another way, thirty-three per cent — one third — of all deaths that occur in people aged less than sixty-five years are attributable to hypertensive causes.

What is Hypertension?

Blood-pressure is measured by the height in millimetres of a column of Mercury that can be raised inside a vacuum. The more pressure there is, the higher the column will rise. Since blood-pressure varies with every heartbeat, two measures are taken — one that measures the pressure of the beat itself (called systolic blood-pressure) and the other that measures the pressure in between beats, when the heart is resting (this is called diastolic blood-pressure, and is the 'background' level). These two figures are written with the systolic figure first followed by the diastolic figure, like this — 120:80.

When we're born, our systolic blood pressure is about forty, then it doubles to about eighty within the first month. Thereafter, the increase is slower, but inexorable, for the rest of our life. Many people do not realize they suffer from hypertension. There may be no symptoms, and it may only be discovered during a visit to the doctor's surgery for another complaint. In its later stages, symptoms may include headache, dizziness, fatigue, and insomnia.

A pressure of 150:90 would be considered above average in a young person, and 160:95 would be abnormally high. In older people, systolic pressure could be 140 at age sixty, and 160 at age eighty years. Comparitively small changes in the pressure of those people who are in the 'at risk' category could have very worthwhile results. This was emphasised by the recent NACNE report, which states:

> It has been estimated that a relatively small reduction (2–3mm) in mean blood-pressure in the population, if the distribution were to remain similar to the present distribution of blood pressures, would result in a major benefit in terms of mortality, and that a shift of this magnitude would be comparable to the benefit currently achieved by antihypertensive therapy. This estimated benefit seems applicable to mild as well as severe hypertension.[4]

If this is true — that a small change in the population's blood-pressure could be as beneficial as all the drugs that people are now taking — then what are we waiting for?

The Pressure is On

Scientists have known for a long time that some populations are apparently 'immune' from hypertension, and do not display the rise in blood pressure that is associated in the West with getting older. These populations generally tend to have a high level of physical activity, are not overweight, have a low level of animal fat in their diet, and don't take much salt (sodium) in their food. In other words, hypertension seems to be an illness of our Western way of life. The problem is, of course, that the majority of us are stuck with it. We can't suddenly emigrate to a tropical paradise, or even change our lifestyles to a significant extent.

As long ago as 1926, it was experimentally shown that certain dietary components could be connected to hypertension. In that year, a pioneering Californian study had shown that the blood-pressure of non-meat using people could be raised — by as much as ten per cent — in just two weeks of eating a diet that is centred around meat.[5] Subsequent experiments have confirmed this effect. Further large-scale studies began to be conducted, and different population groups began to be compared with each other to see just how the variations in diet affected blood-pressure.

One such study was undertaken in Australia.[6] Two groups of people were selected, one of which regularly ate meat in their diets, and the other didn't. Most of the meat-eaters consumed it at least once every day. The non-meat eating group was composed of Australian Seventh Day Adventists. The following graph shows how the two groups compared:

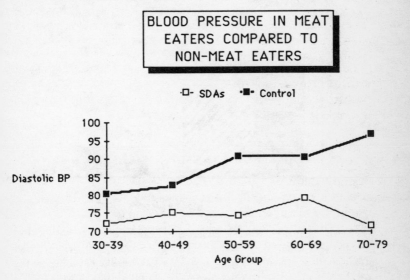

The top line charts the blood-pressure of the meat eaters. The bottom line shows the non-meat eaters, and the bottom axis shows the five age groups that were surveyed. You can see that, at all ages, blood-pressure is significantly lower in the non-meat eaters. Amongst the meat-eaters, there is a steady rise in blood-pressure with advancing age. But amongst the non-meat eaters there is very little increase — and, in fact, a surprising *drop* in blood-pressure in the oldest age group. These results were adjusted to exclude other factors such as exercise, tea or coffee consumption or alcohol.

Another study was carried out in Britain, and again compared the blood-pressure levels in people who didn't eat meat to those who did.[7] The results showed exactly the same pattern. This was true in men as well as women. This chart shows the mean results that were obtained:

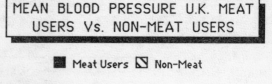

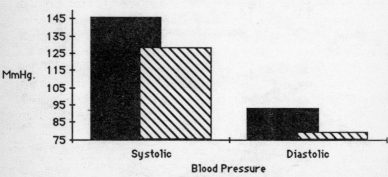

The meat users are shown in black, and non-meat users are shaded. The difference in the 'underlying' blood-pressure (diastolic), which is generally thought to be a better guide to the real health of the individual, is considerable. On average, diastolic blood-pressure was fifteen per cent less in the non-meat users than in the meat-eaters.

Fibre Fans Fight Fat

After the connection between the intake of dietary animal fat and elevated blood-pressure had been established, scientists started looking round for other important dietary factors. It was suggested that a high-fibre diet might somehow give protection against developing high blood-pressure, and from experimental evidence it does seem as if there is some truth in this.

To test this theory, scientists at Southampton University set up an experiment on humans.[8] First, they recruited ninety-four volunteers from the staff and students of the university. Then they divided them into two groups — those who had a high fibre intake in their diets, and those with a low fibre intake. Just as had been expected, the group with the *high* fibre intake had a lower mean blood-pressure than the other group.

The next stage in the experiment was to switch the diets over. So the group who normally ate a high fibre diet was put on a low fibre diet. And the other group was given a diet that was much higher in fibre than the one they had been used to. After four weeks of eating these new diets, the results were measured. Just as you'd expect, the group with the low fibre diet now had *raised* blood-pressure, and the group on high fibre now had *lowered* their blood-pressure. The changes were in the region of five per cent, which is a significant amount. Of course, most meat-oriented diets are essentially low in dietary fibre. Meat itself contains absolutely none.

So it was beginning to look as if a high-meat, low-fibre diet was the worst possible diet for hypertension, particularly when you remember that most meat contains significant quantities of sodium.

Two Further Studies

There is now considerable evidence to show that a meat-free, high-fibre diet can lower blood-pressure, so we will just mention two more. In America, a high plant-fibre diet was devised, including whole-grain cereals, bran cereals, whole-grain breads, vegetables, beans and pulses — but including very little meat or other animal fat.[2] Interestingly, the group put on this diet was allowed to use as much salt in their food as they wanted to. This group was then compared to a standard 'control' group, who carried on eating normally. The average blood-pressure of the men on the plant fibre diet was ten per cent lower than the control group.

The other study we'll briefly mention took place in Australia, where fifty-nine healthy subjects aged twenty-five to sixty-three were randomly allocated to one of three groups.[9] The first was the 'control', which acted as a comparison and continued to eat an ordinary diet for the fourteen weeks that the experiment lasted. The second and third groups were alternately put on a meat-free diet for six weeks each, and then swapped over.

The results revealed a neat pattern. When the first group went on the meatless diet, their blood-pressure dropped significantly. After six weeks, they resumed eating meat, and their blood-pressure went up again. At this point, the second group stopped taking meat, and their pressure dropped, rising again six weeks later when the experiment concluded. The mean changes were 6mmHg (systolic) and 3mmHg (diastolic).

The Possibility of Treatment?

We know — from studies such as those mentioned above — that people on meat-free diets generally exhibit a lower blood-pressure. But could this be used in the treatment of hypertension? Another Australian study tried to do just this.[10]

Fifty-eight people with mild hypertension were selected by scientists at the Royal Perth Hospital. Like the previous study, they were divided into three groups, with the first acting as the 'control' group. Once again, blood pressure fell significantly, by an average of 5mmHg (systolic). The scientists wrote:

> If the usual aim of treatment of mild hypertensives is to reduce systolic blood-pressure to bellow 140mmHg then thirty per cent of those eating a meat-free diet achieved this criteria compared with only eight per cent on their usual diet.

They concluded by suggesting that, if drug therapy was required by a hypertensive, it might also be worthwhile to consider modifying the diet.

One of the most persuasive cases for a meat-free diet to help hypertensives comes from a year-long study in Sweden.[11] In that country, there is an active health movement which claims that a radically altered diet can improve or cure a number of diseases, including hypertension. The experimenters set out to test the claim.

All the twenty-six subjects had a history of high blood pressure, on average for eight years. They were all receiving medication, but even so, eight of the group had excessively high readings (more than 165:95). Many of the patients complained of such symptoms as headache, dizziness, tiredness, and chest pains; symptoms which were either due to the disease or the medication they happened to be taking.

They were then put on a very strict diet indeed. Meat was totally forbidden. So was fish, eggs, milk and milk products. Coffee, tea, sugar, salt and chocolate were also eliminated. They were not allowed to drink chlorinated tap water, but were encouraged to drink natural spring water. Their fresh fruit and vegetables had to be organic, of possible. Despite this, when their diets were analysed, it was found that they were *higher* in vitamins and minerals than most people on a meat diet!

'With the exception of a few essential medicines (for example, insulin),' wrote the scientists, 'patients were encouraged to give up medicines when they felt that these were no longer needed. Thus, analgesics were dispensed with in the absence of pain, tranquillizers when anxiety was not experienced and sleep was sound, and antihypertensive medication when the blood pressure was normal.'

The overall results were indeed impressive. First of all, the patients simply felt much healthier. None of them said that the treatment had left them unchanged or made them feel worse, and fifteen per cent said they felt 'better'. Over fifty per cent of them said they felt 'much better', and thirty per cent said they felt 'completely recovered'.

Actual blood-pressure dropped too, by about six per cent (systolic and diastolic). 'When the decrease in blood-pressure was considered for the entire group,' the scientists wrote, 'it was found that it occurred at the time when most of the medicines were withdrawn. Of the twenty-six patients, twenty had given up their medication completely after one year while six still took some medicine, although the dose was lower, usually halved.'

Several other benefits were found, as well. Their serum cholesterol levels were found to have dropped by an average of fifteen per cent. And the health authorities computed that they had saved about £1,000 per patient over the year, by reducing the costs of drugs and hospitalization.

The Verdict

Hypertension is sometimes prefixed with the word 'essential', which rather confusingly means that the cause is of it is not definitely known to medical science. Nevertheless, we have presented some convincing evidence that implicates meat and other sources of animal fat, while showing that a high plant fibre diet can go some way towards reducing blood pressure. Since hypertension develops so insidiously, and since prevention is the best form of treatment, we should consider the implications of the above evidence when it comes to establishing good long-term eating patterns in our young children. For those people who have already developed hypertension, it would seem to make sense to investigate the serious possibility of dietary modification following the example of the Swedish experiment.

REFERENCES

1. 'Plant Fiber and Blood Pressure', J. W. Anderson, *Annals of Internal Medicine* 1983:98. 842-846.
2. 'Does a Vegetarian Diet reduce the Occurrence of Diabetes?', D. A. Snowdon, R. L. Phillips, *American Journal of Public Health* 1985; 75:507–512.
3. Mortality Statistics: Cause (1978) HMSO 1980.
4. 'Proposals for nutritional guidelines for health education in Britain',

The Health Education Council, National Advisory Committee on Nutrition Education, September 1983.

5. 'The relation of protein foods to hypertension', A. N. Donaldson, *Californian and Western Medicine*, 1926:24,328.

6. 'Blood Pressure in Seventh day Adventist Vegetarians', B. Armstrong, A. J. Van Merwyk, H. Coates, *American Journal of Epidemiology*, Vol. 105, no. 5.

7. 'Haemostatic variables in vegetarians and non-vegetarians', A. P. Haines, R. Chakrabarti, D. Fisher, T. W. Meade, W. R. S. North, Y. Stirling, *Thrombosis Research* 19; 139–148, 1980.

8. 'Dietary fibre and blood-pressure', A. Wright, P. G. Burstyn, M. J. Gibney, *British Medical Journal*, 15 December 1979.

9. 'Blood-pressure-lowering effect of a vegetarian diet: controlled trial in normotensive subjects', I. L. Rouse, B. K. Armstrong, L. J. Beilen, R. Vandongen, '*The Lancet*', 1 January 1983.

10. 'A randomized control trial of a vegetarian diet in the treatment of mild hypertension', B. M. Margetts, L. J. Beilin, B. K. Armstrong, R. Vandongen, *Clininal and Experimental Pharmacology and Physiology*, (1985) 12, 263–266.

11. 'A vegan regime with reduced medication in the treatment of hypertension', O. Lindahl, L. Lindwall, A. Spångberg, Å. Stenram, P. A. Öckerman, *British Journal of Nutrition* (1984), 52, 11–20.

9

How to Get High on Fibre

Are you constipated at the moment?

Four people out of every ten in the United Kingdom will answer 'yes' to that question (assuming they're not too embarrassed to mention the subject). In twenty per cent of the population, constipation is so severe that laxatives are used regularly.

Let's get down to the bottom line.

It's an amazing (but true) fact that seventy-seven per cent of the population only excrete between five and seven stools per week. *Over three quarters of the total population*! On top of that, a further eight per cent of people only pass three to four stools a week. That makes eighty-five per cent of us with slow bowel movements.[1] No wonder the laxative manufacturers are making record profits. But what is the cause of this massive go-slow?

In a word — fibre, or rather, the lack of it in our diets. Everyone's heard about fibre — in fact, you can't escape from it at the moment. They won't *let* you escape from it. Everywhere you look — television, posters, magazines — they're all trying to sell you fibre. You can buy specially formulated 'high-fibre' pills from the chemist, and even the sickliest breakfast cereal now features 'added fibre'. Fibre has become Big Business, which is not surprising considering the enormous size of the potential market.

But although most people have heard about fibre, not many actually understand what it is, how they get it, how much they need, and what it really does to them. That's why they're getting such a bum deal. For this state of affairs, we have to blame the advertisers, who are keener to sell you their latest 'high-fibre' product than they are to ensure that you have an *understanding* of the nature of fibre in a healthy diet. One problem that the manufacturers don't mention, for example, is the difference between a product that features 'added fibre', and another product that may not have 'specially added fibre'. Which product is the healthier and best for you? It's not easy for consumers to decide, because they're bombarded with so much propaganda. The answer is that the product that features 'added fibre' *may not* be the best for you. Because you should aim to get your dietary fibre primarily from natural sources, and not from artificially-concocted products. This is how the NACNE report explained it:

> It is suggested that dietary fibre might best be derived from foods, and not from either dietary fibre preparations or foods to which bran and other fibres have been added. By not advocating foods to which fibres are specifically added one is more likely to ensure that the whole grain product will be used and this is more likely to ensure increased intakes of minerals, trace elements and other micronutrients; elemental malabsorption is also then less likely.[1]

So you should forget about the commercial 'added-fibre' foods and concentrate on finding natural food sources of fibre. One way to achieve this is to cut out or cut down on your meat consumption. Automatically, your natural fibre consumption will tend to increase.

This happens because meat contains absolutely no fibre. It is therefore useless from the point of view of supplying our essential dietary fibre. But there is also a further problem with a meat-orientated diet. Because meat is a very heavy, dense food, it tends to fill you up quickly. It is a very concentrated form of calories, most of them coming from fat. So when you've eaten meat, you no longer *feel* like eating bulkier (but lighter) plant food. Meat therefore acts to minimize the intake of dietary fibre in two ways.

What is Dietary Fibre?

Imagine a honeycomb, with the honey separated by an intricate structure of wax cells. It looks rather like the way that plants organize their own cells, except they're much smaller. In a plant, the cell structure is made from fibre, not wax. Dietary fibre is, essentially, the cell-wall material of plants. The 'honeycomb' comparison is actually quite a good one, because one of the fibre's functions is to 'lock up' the nutrients (i.e. the honey) in the cells, until they are required. In Figure 1, you can see that the carbohydrate in the cell is completely enclosed by fibre (thick black outline).

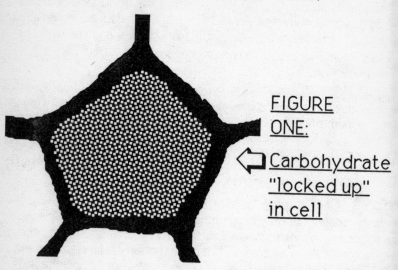

<u>FIGURE ONE:</u>

⇐ <u>Carbohydrate "locked up" in cell</u>

Another of fibre's functions is to 'stiffen' the plant — it acts like nature's scaffolding. This is what makes plant food chewy. When we cook, mill or process our food in some other way, what we are basically doing is to reduce the strength of this 'scaffolding', so that we can eat it more easily and also to 'unlock' some of the nutrients that the fibre wraps up. This is one of the objections to some of the processes of our modern food industry — that it destroys the fibre to such an extent that the micronutrients it encloses are exposed and destroyed. That's why just adding a cup full of fibre (e.g. bran) to a low fibre diet isn't as good as eating *natural* fibre foods. All you're doing by adding fibre is to eat the wrapping paper — without getting to the present!

There's another problem with eating processed food, too. Figure 2 shows the same plant cell as before, but this time after it's been milled and turned into white flour. As you can see, most of the fibre has been destroyed, and the carbohydrate is now much more accessible.

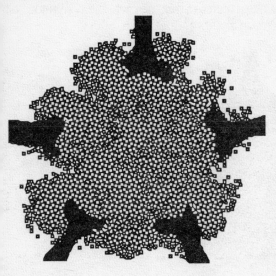

FIGURE TWO: Refined Carbohydrate (White Flour)

However, in something like white sugar (or even brown sugar, or molasses) there is *no* fibre left at all. This is shown in Figure 3. Here, all the carbohydrate (mainly in the form of sucrose) can be *immediately* absorbed by the body, without having to break down any of the fibrous barriers, because the processing has already taken care of it. This can present a serious problem to the body. Eating this sort of food creates an instant rise in the blood sugar level, followed by a sharp drop again as the body tries to set things back in balance. But our bodies simply aren't adjusted to take in sudden and massive doses of 'instant energy'. They're much happier when they've got some *unrefined* carbohydrate (i.e. complete with some fibre) to work on. This way, the body can slowly release just the right amount of energy when we need it. It's a very sophisticated process, which has developed through our evolution to handle a natural diet of fibre-rich foods, and it has worked extremely well for tens of thousands of years. Yet, only in the past 100 years, we have managed to completely upset this delicate process by stripping most of the fibre away from our natural foods, and at the same time drastically increasing the amount of animal fat in our diet. The combination couldn't have been worse.

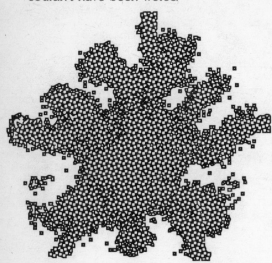

FIGURE THREE: Refined Carbohydrate (Sugar)

Carbohydrate Rules O.K.

We've mentioned carbohydrates, so maybe it would be a good idea to go over a few points about them. Firstly, carbohydrates are one of three principle sources of energy for the body (the other two are fats and protein). There are three basic types of carbohydrates:

1. *Sugars*: Both simple and double sugars, such as honey, table sugar, and the sugar found in fruits, are very quickly and easily absorbed by the body.

2. *Starches*: These are chains of simple sugars, which need the body's enzyme action to break them down. Found in grains, legumes, vegetables.

3. *Cellulose*: This, quite simply, is what we call 'fibre'.

The essence of modern food processing is 'refining', which means separating the fibre from the other carbohydrate that is naturally found in plants. Sugar cane, for example, is refined to produce table sugar. And wheat (unrefined carbohydrate) is processed to produce white flour (refined carbohydrate), in the process exposing its micronutrients to degradation and throwing away most of the valuable fibre. White bread today contains virtually no fibre.

Enter the 'Saccharine Disease'

Over the past hundred years, one or two individuals have raised their voices to warn people about the dangers of eating a highly processed, over-refined diet. No-one listened to them, of course. Then, in the mid-1950s, some scientists began to formulate a hypothesis for a collection of illnesses they termed the 'Saccharine Disease'. They argued that there were two main dangers from eating such a highly refined diet. Firstly, it meant that people were consuming highly-concentrated food that was too quick and easy to eat — as a result, they were getting fatter and obese. This new obesity increased the body's demand for the hormone insulin to deal with all the extra blood sugar, leading to a continuing rise in the number of diabetics. The other danger, they believed, was a result of the sheer lack of fibre, which was invariably thrown away during food processing. It was suggested, for the first time, that this fibre *might* have a more important role in the prevention of disease than simply being easily discarded 'wrapping paper'.

High Meat Means Low Fibre

As we've already mentioned, meat itself contains no fibre. But apart from that, the level of meat in the diet has been found to be directly proportional to the lack of fibre — the more meat you eat, the less fibre you're likely to get. A fascinating experiment, comparing data gathered from Western and African countries showed just how this relationship works.

Dr Denis Burkitt, a famous advocate of dietary fibre, collected information from various populations concerning the size of their stools, the average time it took food to pass all the way through their bodies, and the type of diet they ate.[2] You can see some of his results in the following chart.

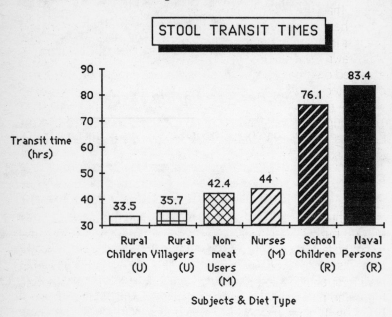

STOOL TRANSIT TIMES

Transit time (hrs)

Rural Children (U)	Rural Villagers (U)	Non-meat Users (M)	Nurses (M)	School Children (R)	Naval Persons (R)
33.5	35.7	42.4	44	76.1	83.4

Subjects & Diet Type

His findings were very exciting indeed. From left to right on the chart, the first group, with the shortest 'stool transit time', were schoolchildren living in rural Africa, eating an unrefined diet. Their food positively shot through their insides, taking on average less than a day and a half from one end to the other. Next came another group of Africans, this time adults living in villages in Uganda. Once again, their food hardly touched the sides on the way down.

But it is the next group that is so interesting from our point of view. This consisted not of Africans, eating a natural diet, but of ordinary people living in the United Kingdom, leading normal lives, *but not eating meat*. Despite enormous differences in environment and food availability, the similarity between the U.K. non-meat users diet and the natural African one is very striking.

The next group on the chart consisted of Indian nurses living and working in South India. Once again, their diet would tend towards the meat-free, and their transit times were only slightly longer than the U.K. non-meat users.

But then the really big jump comes. The next group has nearly twice as long a transit time as any of the preceding ones. This group was drawn from children at a boarding school in the U.K., eating a refined diet typical of institutionalized catering — greasy, meat-dominated, and low in natural fibre. And the next group is even worse — naval ratings and their wives, all shore-based in the U.K. This group had a mean transit time of 83.4 hours, and the longest time was 144 hours. That's six whole days for the food to hang around someone's intestines!

Big, Fast and Regular!

You might suppose that small stools would whizz through the system quickly, but you'd be wrong. For Burkitt found that the larger the stool, the faster it was processed. So, for example, the mean weight of stools passed by naval ratings was a mere 104 grams (not even 4 ounces), and certainly nothing to write home about. On the other hand, the mean weight for rural Ugandan villagers was a mind-boggling 470 grams. Just over a pound!

Somewhere in the middle came the U.K. non-meat users, with a mean weight of 225 grams (8 ounces), who compare very favourably with South African schoolchildren (275grams/9 ounces) and Indian nurses (155 grams/5 ounces).

The Significance of the Results

This information was crucial to our understanding of the importance of a natural fibre diet. Further evidence has shown that, without exception, countries which have a refined diet in which meat is predominant face a whole range of diseases that less 'advanced' countries rarely see. Some of these diseases, which can be directly associated to the western, high-meat and fat, low-fibre diet include:

- *Appendicitis* is the commonest abdominal emergency in the West. Over 300,000 appendixes are removed every year in the United States alone. It has now been experimentally proven that a low-fibre diet makes the risk of suffering appendicitis much greater.
- *Diverticular disease* is a swelling, with possible infection and complications, of the colon, and thirty per cent of all people over forty-five years have symptoms.
- *Cancer of the Large Bowel* is, after lung cancer, the most common cause of death from cancer in the West.

But these diseases were all comparitively rare, in the United Kingdom, until the beginning of the twentieth century. Then the

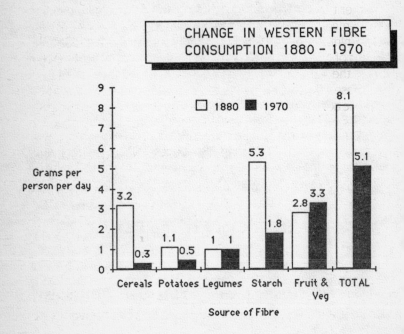

CHANGE IN WESTERN FIBRE CONSUMPTION 1880 – 1970

Grams per person per day

☐ 1880 ■ 1970

Source of Fibre	1880	1970
Cereals	3.2	0.3
Potatoes	1.1	0.5
Legumes	1	1
Starch	5.3	1.8
Fruit & Veg	2.8	3.3
TOTAL	8.1	5.1

amount of animal fat in the diet began to steadily increase, and the amount of raw natural fibre began to decrease. This is how the American diet has changed in less than 100 years — the picture in Britain is much the same.

A hundred years ago meat, fat and sugar between them only contributed fifteen per cent of the total amount of calories in the diet. Today, the figure is nearer sixty per cent. Perhaps the biggest change in the diet has been the tremendous fall in the quantity of cereal fibre, which has dropped by ninety per cent. Most scientists now accept that there is a definite connection between the diseases mentioned above and the radical change in our eating patterns. It is not altogether certain how the relationship works, and it may take many years to find out scientifically. One theory, for example, is that carcinogens and mutagens (such as nitrosamines found in meat) are being exposed to our intestines in much larger quantities and for longer periods (i.e. transit times) than ever before, and this certainly could be one avenue of promising research.

Another theory concerning cancer of the colon again features the high-meat/low fibre dietary relationship. In this theory, the high level of animal fat in the diet causes the liver to secrete considerable amounts of bile acids. Then, the raised fat level alters the bacteria living in the gut — some are killed off, and some new ones take over. These newly-active bacteria get to work with their enzymes on the bile acid, and decompose it to form various cancer-producing chemicals. Now normally, these chemicals would be absorbed by natural fibre. But in this high-meat/low-fibre diet, there's just not enough fibre to go round. So the carcinogens hang around in the intestines for a prolonged period until they are finally expelled in the stools. But in the meantime, of course, our bodies have been exposed to more cancer-causing substances. Once again, this illustrates the strong connection between eating too much flesh food and not enough plant food. Quite plainly, it's out of balance.

Gallstones — Being Kicked in the Guts by a Steak

Gallstones are a very common complaint, and can frequently be excruciatingly painful. One sufferer compared it to 'being kicked in the guts by a horse — all the time.' But if any animals are involved in this complaint, it's more likely to be the ones we eat. Because there is now evidence to associate the occurrence of gallstones with a low-fibre, high-meat diet.

Gallstones are mainly composed of solidified cholesterol. They can be formed in the gall bladder, where they can stay quite happily for years. However, they can also lead to infection, resulting in inflamation of the gall bladder, colic, peritonitis, gangrene of the gall bladder, and jaundice. They are more common amongst women than men — twenty-five per cent of all women and ten per cent of all men will develop gallstones before they are sixty years old. The obese and diabetic are also more at risk.

It is likely that there is a strong metabolic connection in the development of gallstones. The liver secretes bile, a substance that is high in cholesterol (which literally means 'solid bile' in Greek), and is stored in the gall bladder. Lecithin (found in soya beans and corn) and bile salts together help to keep the cholesterol dissolved in the bile. However, if the level of cholesterol becomes so high that no more can be dissolved, then it begins to precipitate, and gallstones are the result.

Almost half of all those people with gallstones feel no symptoms. If a stone obstructs a passage, however, pain will be felt in the abdomen, with nausea and vomiting, particularly after eating fatty food. Sometimes cholesterol will be precipitated so heavily that it is deposited around the body, especially in the eyelids. It is known that overweight people have a greater risk of suffering from gallstones. Orientals and rural Africans, who traditionally consume a low-fat, low cholesterol, high-fibre diet, suffer very little from them. In addition, only humans and domesticated animals have gallstones, wild animals do not. This also tends to suggest that the problem is connected with our modern, Western lifestyle.

In an experiment carried out in Oxford, England, two groups of women were compared to see if their diets could have any influence on the occurrence of gallstones.[3] The first group, consisting of 632 women, were selected at random, and ate meat. The second group consisted of 130 women who did not eat meat, and had a diet naturally higher in fibre. All the women were then given a thorough inspection, using ultrasound detection techniques, looking specifically for gallstones. The experimenters found that the meat-eaters were *two and a half times* more likely to develop gallstones than the non-meat eaters. The scientists concluded that the low-fat, high-fibre diet of the non-meat eating women gave them protection.

What You Need and Where to Get it

According to the government's NACNE report, we should increase the fibre content of our diet by a full fifty per cent, from twenty grams per day up to thirty grams. A heavy meat diet delivers little fibre but provides fats and other highly concentrated sources of calories that we don't need. By substituting cereals, vegetables and fruit for meat and meat products we can *cut out* a product that we don't have a biological need for, and *replace* it with one for which we do have a proven need. What sort of food should you eat? Here is a list of some popular foods with their fibre contents:

Food	Measure	Fibre (g)
Chickpeas	1 cup	10
Pinto Beans	1 cup	8
Millet	1 cup	7.3
Whole Wheat Pita Bread	1 average	6
Blackberries	1 cup	5.9
Dried Figs	5 medium	5.6
Sunflower Seeds	1 cup	5.5
Wheat Bran	1 cup	5.2
Nori	100g	4.7
Red Currants	1 cup	4.5
Azuki Beans	1 cup	4.3
Brazil Nuts	1 cup	4.2
Dried Apricot	1 cup	3.9
Almonds	1 cup	3.8
Peanuts	1 cup	3.8

Food	Measure	Fibre (g)
Avocado	1 raw	3.2
Peas	1 cup	3
Gooseberries	1 cup	2.9
Whole Wheat Flour	1 cup	2.8
Wheat Germ	1 cup	2.5
Whole Wheat Bread	1 slice	2.5
Lentils	1 cup	2.4
Rice	1 cup	2.4
Broccoli	1 cup	2
Soya Flour	1 cup	2
Cornflakes	1 cup	2
Carrots	1 cup	1.5
Baked Potato	1 large	1.2
Onion	1 cup	1
Celery	1 cup	0.7

REFERENCES

1. 'Proposals for nutritional guidelines for health education in Britain', The Health Education Council, National Advisory Committee on Nutrition Education, September 1983.
2. 'Effect of dietary Fibre on stools and transit times, and its role in the causation of disease, D. P. Burkitt, A. R. P. Walker, N. S. Painter, *The Lancet*, 30 December 1972.
3. 'Effect of vegetarianism on development of gallstones in women', F. Pixley, D. Wilson, K. McPherson, J. Mann, *British Medical Journal*, Vol. 291, 7 July 1985.

10

A View into Hell

My friend looked rather guilty as he diffidently chewed on his hamburger. He'd been talking to me about the pro's and con's of a meat-free diet, a subject that he'd raised himself. Then he came out with a remark that I'd heard hundreds of times before.

'Of course,' he said, 'I wouldn't eat meat if I had to kill the cow myself.'

He spoke half-apologetically, almost as if he felt he had to put forward some kind of excuse. I felt embarrassed for him, and awkward too. I didn't want to endorse his remark too enthusiastically, in case he got the impression I was trying to be 'holier-than-thou'. On the other hand, I couldn't disagree with him. Because he'd spoken the truth — a truth that all people who still eat animal flesh somehow have to come to terms with.

The way that the majority of people come to terms with this problem is simply to ignore it, and pretend that it just doesn't exist. After all, killing an animal cannot be described as a pleasant business, so it is not surprising if the majority of us choose to delegate the whole objectionable process to an anonymous slaughterman in a distant slaughterhouse, as far away from our own sensibilities as possible. And we're actually encouraged to do this by the meat industry. *They* don't want our consciences troubled — it's bad for business. This fact was highlighted recently in the following news report:

The editor in chief of the *Meat Trades Journal* today urged that the words 'butcher' and 'slaughterhouse' be eradicated and replaced by the American euphemisms 'meat plant' or 'meat factory'. Alternatively, butchers could adopt the Irish word 'victualler'. This would distance consumers from awareness of the 'bloodier side' of the meat trade. The editor argued that it was time for a review of meat trade vocabulary in recognition of 'a growing away among younger meat buyers from the concept that meat ever comes from an animal.' This was partly because these buyers did their shopping in the bloodless ambiance of supermarkets. The meat trade's cause was not helped by the 'blood-spattered whites' of Smithfield porters as they strolled 'in front of the secretary birds.' They and butchers should be put into velvet overalls. 'It will reduce cleaning bills and any adverse reaction from the fainthearted.' These days the word 'butcher' was spread over newspaper headlines about the Ripper or the aftermath of bomb attacks. A change of nomenclature might only seem a verbal difference but it would 'conjure up an image of meat divorced from the act of slaughter.' 'The public does not want to be made aware of the bloodier side of slaughter,' he said. 'Perhaps now is the time for changes to be made.'[1]

You could argue, of course, that the public is perfectly entitled to not want to know what happens to their meat before it lands up on their plate. This point was made to me once by a radio interviewer.

'I go to the toilet without thinking about sewage works', he said. 'I find sewage works offensive, and I have no desire to ever see one. But that doesn't make me a hypocrite each time I go to the toilet, does it?'

'Ah,' I replied, 'there are several important differences. For a start, *everyone* has to go to the toilet. But eating meat is strictly optional — people do it just for pleasure, it's not an essential requirement. And as far as I'm concerned, any pleasure that I got from eating meat would be vastly outweighed by the suffering I would have inflicted on other living creatures.'

'There's another point, too,' I continued. 'When children are small, we try to teach them to be responsible for themselves. That means honestly facing up to and accepting the consequences of their actions. By paying other people — slaughtermen in this case — to do our 'dirty work' for us, we're neither being responsible nor truly honest with ourselves. If you can't face the thought of an animal leading a miserable life, and dying a painful death just for your own appetite, then there's really only one decision you can responsibly come to.'

Some vets — and cooks — are of the opinion that it is possible to detect those animals which suffer agonizing deaths by the taste of the meat itself. One vet says that the 'bolts' of tough meat encountered in carcasses is due solely to the massive shock suffered by the animal. Certainly, the slaughtering industry tries very hard to artificially 'tenderize' the meat by a variety of methods, including enzyme injections into the live animal. This is what one famous cook says about meat that comes from animals which have suffered fear or pain before death:

> Quite definitely, trapped, hurt or slowly-killed animals are bad food. One example will serve: if you see a rabbit for sale with bloody, crushed legs, your own intelligence will tell you that it has been trapped and held in agony for hours, and should never be eaten. Intelligent women will refuse to buy rabbit, hare or any game that has been cut up so the method of killing has been disguised. For in meat killed in high fever, the bloodstream is charged with glandular secretions and unfit for human consumption.[2]

But in today's modern butcher's shop, it is quite impossible to tell if the animal was in extreme agony before it died. Unfortunately, all the evidence that comes from the dark world of the slaughterhouse indicates that most animals *do* suffer horrific fates.

Into the Darkness

It is becoming increasingly difficult to gain access to slaughter-houses. No-one wants outsiders there (particularly not any media), to witness and report the many shortcomings that exist. Sometimes, usually through subterfuge, outsiders *do* get in. Here are three accounts by outside observers of what they saw. They are straightforward and unsensational accounts, which perhaps makes them all the more horrifying.

> Before we went in, our guide, the manager of the place, gave us a short

description of what we would see. We then went in, and the things that immediately struck us were the noise (mainly mechanical) and the awful stench.

The first thing we saw was the cattle being killed. They came one by one from the holding pens, up an alleyway into a high sided metal pen. A man leaned over with a captive bolt pistol, and shot them between the eyes. This stunned them and they fell down. The side of the pen then lifted up and the cow rolled out on its side. The cow appeared to be completely rigid, as if every muscle in its body was tensed. The same man put a chain round the cow's hock and electrically winched it up into the air until just its head was resting on the flour. He then got a large piece of wire (we were told it was not electrified) and stuck it into the hole that the pistol had made. We were told that this killed the cow by severing the connection between its brain and its spinal cord. Every time the man inserted the wire into a cow's brain the animal kicked out and struggled even though it was apparently unconscious. Several times while we were watching this operation, the cow fell from the pen kicking as it had not been properly stunned, and the man had to use the pistol on it again.

Once the cow was dead it was winched right up so that its head was about two to three feet off the flour. It was then moved round to a man who slit its throat. When he did this a torrent of blood poured out, splashing everywhere including all over us. He also cut the forelegs off at the knee. Then another man cut off the head which was put on one side. Then the hide was removed by a man who was standing up high on a platform, and then the carcass moved on again to where the whole body was split open, and all the lungs, stomach, intestines etc came flopping out. We were horrified on a couple of occasions to see a fairly large, well-developed calf come out as well, as the cow had been in a late stage of pregnancy. Our guide told us that this was a regular occurrence.

The carcass was then split into two by a man who sawed it down the spine with a short of chain saw, and then the case was ready for cold store. While we were there only cattle were being 'processed' but there were sheep waiting in the holding pens. The animals that were waiting to be killed showed obvious signs of extreme fear — panting, staring eyes and frothing at the mouth. We were told that the sheep and pigs were killed by electrocution, but this method could not be used on cattle as it required such a high voltage to kill, that the blood would separate and the meat would look as it if were full of black dots.[3]

Here is another eyewitness account of the same process, witnessed this time by representatives of the media.

> In the holding pens the slaughtermen were trying to move a young but fully-grown steer. The animal could sense and smell the death before him and didn't want to move. Using prods and spikes they drove him forwards and into a special restraint where he received a meat tenderizing injection. A few minutes later the animal was driven reluctantly into the stunning box and the gate slammed shut. He was then 'stunned' by a captive bolt pistol, his legs buckled beneath him, the gate was opened, and he sprawled out onto the floor. They pushed a wire into the half-inch diameter puncture made in his forehead by the stun bolt and twisted it. He kicked whilst the wire was in and then was still. A chain shackle was put around one of his hind legs, at which point he started struggling and kicking whilst he was hoisted over the blood bath. He was then still. A slaughterman then approached with a knife. Many people saw the steer's eyes focus on the slaughterman and follow him as he approached. He struggled both before and as the knife went in. The universal opinion, including that of the press, was that this was *not* a reflex action — he was conscious and struggling. The knife was inserted twice and he bled into the bath.

And finally, here is an account of everyday death in a municipal slaughterhouse, whose operations are heavily subsidized by the local ratepayers. The first type of slaughter described is that undertaken for 'religious' reasons, and legally takes place without any requirement for pre-stunning, meaning that animal is fully conscious while it bleeds to death.

> Ritual slaughter was first. The sheep are brought in one at a time (or three at a time, if nobody's looking) and placed, back down, on a low table. Their throats are then sliced with a sharp knife whilst their back leg is being shackled; then, up the hoist to bleed to death. This, of course, is assuming that the first cut works. Otherwise the slaughterman finds himself with a fight on his hands as the sheep rolls round the floor in agony in its own blood. These sheep are 'awkward buggers' or 'stupid bastards' because they don't want to be killed.
>
> Electrocution of pigs I found particularly distressing. After their pitiful

life of confinement they are rushed down the motorway to their fate. Their night in the lairage is probably the most comfortable they have ever spent. Here they have sawdust bedding and are fed and watered. But this brief glimpse of daylight is to be their last. The squeals as they succumb to the electric stunner is one of the most pathetic sounds imaginable. The photographer stood by taking photos, whilst the slaughterman looked to us for sympathy. 'You don't want to be watching this, this is easy work. You should have seen the big boar we had in here yesterday. They can do you a real injury, they can.'[4]

Just Some of the Problems

Many Official Veterinary Surgeons (O.V.S.s) will admit (in private) that conditions for the animals they are supposed to be responsible for are often far from ideal. And yet there seems to be nothing that anyone is prepared to do to improve things. I spoke to many O.V.S.s while researching this book and was frequently shocked by what they told me. One of them even admitted to me that he deliberately tried not to visit slaughterhouses more often than he had to — he found the conditions too disturbing, and felt powerless to do anything about them.

'One of the main problems', an O.V.S. told me, 'is the total lack of training available to slaughtermen. There is no legal requirement for them to be trained at all. All the law says is that they have to be over eighteen, and a 'fit and proper person', whatever that may mean.'

'But they have to be licensed, don't they?', I objected.

'The licensing arrangements are a complete disgrace,' the vet said. 'The local authority is responsible for giving them — it's not up to trained vets like me, although we probably know more about the process than anyone else, and we are certainly more expert than whoever it is in the local authority who sends out the licences. The real scandal, however, is that the authority never *refuses* or takes away anyone's licence. So any sadist can apply, and he'll get his licence, with no fuss at all. There has never been a case of a slaughterman's licence being withdrawn.'

'What other problems are there?' I asked him.

'The men become very hard,' he said. 'After just a week or two working in the slaughterhouse, they're quite desensitized, if that's the right expression. I've often seen it happen. They soon forget they're dealing with animals. The cruelty isn't always intentional, but the animals still suffer unnecessarily. One of the causes of this is the way they're paid. They're usually on piece-work, which means the more animals they kill the more they get paid. This is a big problem in all the main slaughterhouses, where thousands of animals may be killed each week.'

'So what happens when a mistake is made?' I asked.

'Some of the worst things happen when new slaughtermen are trying to learn how to do the job. Animals are frequently not stunned properly, so they're still alive during the next stages of processing. It annoys me that even experienced slaughtermen still don't understand that just because an animal may have fallen over, it may not be unconscious. This happens a lot to pigs. They're supposed to be stunned by a pair of electric tongs that must be held on its head for at least seven seconds, until the animal has a fit. But you're dealing here with a frightened, squealing animal. It won't stand still and wait to be killed. Sometimes the tongs slips and go into the pig's eye, which is very nasty. Sometimes the tongs are blocked up with burnt hair and skin, so not much current goes through.'

'The worst thing,' he continued, 'is that supposedly experienced slaughtermen will just use the tongs to immobilize the pigs with — they don't see why they should waste time and hold them on the pig's head for seven seconds. And, although they're not supposed to, they still stun a batch of five or six pigs at a time before going on to cut their throats and bleed them out. I've frequently seen the first one or two pigs in a batch start to recover consciousness before the last ones have been stunned. But it doesn't seem to bother the men.'

'Why don't they just kill the animals outright, and very quickly?' I asked him.

'I wish they would,' he replied. 'But there's a strong myth in the meat industry that an animal's heart must be beating while the blood is draining out through the jugular cut. It's supposed to get rid of more, and so improve the meat. It's totally untrue, and has been proven to be so. Even though an animal's heart may still be beating, you can't drain all the blood away. That's why they're supposed to stun them first, without killing them.'

A gruesome thought struck me. 'What happens to all the blood?' I enquired.

'Down the drains,' he said. 'About half of it is poured straight down the drain, the rest goes for pet food.'

'How often do you visit each slaughterhouse?' I asked.

'On average, we have the resources to visit each one about once every six months. That's for slaughterhouses killing for the domestic market. For the export market, there must be a vet present most of the time. The public just don't know that there two, very different, standards operating in this country.'

'Which animals do you think are the most badly treated?' I asked.

'There's no doubt in my mind that poultry gets the worst deal. A battery hen leads a hell of a life. No-one seems to think that birds can suffer as much as other animals. A lot of the big poultry processing plants are very automated, and they suffer there, too. The problem with chickens is that they're not all the same standard size. But the machinery is only set to handle an "average" bird. After they're hung by their feet on the processing line, they're supposed to go through a electrified water dip that stuns them. But the big ones and the little ones aren't stunned. So they can go alive into the scalding tanks. I've seen this happen. You can always tell when a bird has gone in alive, because it comes out the other end a bright pink colour. They're always thrown away, those ones don't end up on the supermarket shelves.'

No Interest, No Concern, No Action

The most damning piece of 'official' evidence against the slaughtering business that has yet been produced is the Farm Animal Welfare Council's 'Report on the Welfare of Livestock at the Time of Slaughter'. This, according to Britain's R.S.P.C.A., is a 'massive indictment of the way that food animals are slaughtered'.

The Farm Animal Welfare Council (F.A.W.C.) is a quasi-official organization, set up in 1979 by the Ministry of Agriculture; yet held at a suitably discreet distance from the Ministry itself. It's role is purely advisory; whether the officials at the Ministry, or even the Minister himself, accepts, rejects, or (as at the moment) ignores their advice is not up to the F.A.W.C.

Their report produced fifty-one recommendations for legislation, eleven for better enforcement, twenty-five for a code of practice, nine for research, fourteen for design, and seven general recommendations.

So far, *not one* has resulted in stricter legislation or controls. Here are some of the major concerns the report expresses:

Money Comes First: The inquiry found that the slaughtering industry was 'suffering considerable economic problems'. These commercial considerations, they felt, was contributing to the overlooking of welfare needs, which the report 'deplored'.

No Powers of Enforcement: The responsibility for enforcing both hygiene and animal welfare in slaughterhouses rests with local authorities. The report found that 'in many cases local authorities are not taking their responsibilities seriously enough, nor is it clear where overall responsibility lies within their organization.' This means that there is often no effective control exercized in either of these areas.

Bad Design: They found that welfare problems were exacerbated by poor design of the slaughtering premises, and it was 'of considerable concern that such faults were often to be found in modern, purpose-built premises.' The problems included lack of space for animals waiting to be slaughtered, no ventilation or watering facilities, and slippery floors. 'Little account appeared to have been taken of the welfare needs,' the report said.

Cruelty During Unloading: They found that such legislation that exists was not being properly enforced by local authorities, leading to animals slipping and falling from ramps and damaging themselves in other ways as they are herded through. They saw slaughtermen using 'electric goads', stick-like devices that deliver a painful electric shock, when trying to unload frightened animals. 'In many cases,' they found, 'the use of an electric goad was counter-productive, creating confusion and stress for the animal,' and they also saw 'too many cases of random application of electric goads to the head and shoulders and instances of stick abuse to the anal or genital area of the animal.'

Terror Before Killing: Cattle were found to be particularly stressed prior to slaughter, 'baulking at the approach, and this all too often resulted in the excessive use of goads; the noise of the slaughterhall activity, together with the banging of the side and rear gates of the metal-sheeted box, will deter them from entering and, once encased in the box, they are trapped in a noisy and very strange environment — in some cases for several minutes while hold-ups on the slaughter line ahead are being cleared. In our view such handling arrangements prior to stunning often create a high level of stress, even terror, for the animals.' They also reported instances of animals being confined in the killing stall for five minutes or more, in sheer terror, just waiting to be killed.

The report goes on to make many more points. It is, perhaps, one of the biggest *official* indictments of the brutal and callous way that we treat the animals that we intend to land up on someone's dinner plate. Sadly, it is overly-optimistic to think that any significant change will result from it. To change, to improve the welfare of these animals will cost the industry money. And who cares? As one slaughterman said, 'What's the point in treating them well? They're going to die in any case, aren't they?'

An Obscene Ritual

Religious slaughter — or ritual slaughter, as it is more popularly known — is not purely the concern of the Muslims and Jews who believe it to be necessary. It is actually the responsibility of us all. Because every person who eats meat will, without knowing, have eaten ritually slaughtered food at some time.

It's estimated that seventy per cent of the meat that comes from animals which have been killed by ritual means actually ends up on the open market, finding its way into everyone's school meals, restaurants, and meat products of all descriptions. Britain is now a major exporter of ritually-slaughtered meat to Europe and the Middle East. But what exactly *is* ritual slaughter?

One vet I spoke to described it as the most revolting sight he had ever seen inside a slaughterhouse. The process does not allow pre-stunning of the animal, so that it is fully conscious while it bleeds. He told me how he saw four slaughtermen holding one sheep down on the slaughtering table — the animals struggle so much that it usually takes several men to pin them down. The slaughterer then cuts the animal's neck open, and allows it to bleed to death. 'He didn't cut so much as saw', the vet said to me. 'It took four attempts by the slaughterman before the animal's arteries were finally severed.' When the animal has weakened sufficiently, it is hung up and left to die.

Ritual slaughter is demanded by certain Muslims and Jews, who believe it to be an important part of their religious principles. For this reason, critics of ritual slaughter are sometimes accused of being racially-motivated. In defence of the practice, its proponents claim that the loss of blood the animal suffers is so sudden that it induces rapid unconsciousness. This is how the Chairman of the Schechita Committee of the board of Deputies of British Jews explains it:

> The animal's throat is cut, and the whole operation can, if done properly, take less than half a minute. People imagine that because the animal has its throat cut while fully conscious it must be in pain. But what has been found as a result of experiments conducted in the late 1970s at the University of Hanover is that the animal becomes unconscious within two seconds of its throat being cut.[5]

Still Conscious After Stunning: They saw baby calves, after having supposedly been stunned, being suspended upside down on the bleeding line, with their throats cut, *still* bleating. This they found 'distressing', although they couldn't state scientifically that the calves were conscious. 'We have concluded,' they reported, 'that unconsciousness and insensibility are being assumed to exist in many slaughtering operations when it is highly probable that the degree is not sufficient to render the animal insensitive to pain.'

Stunning that Doesn't Work: They found considerable evidence that slaughtermen were unable to produce a quick and clean kill. If a pistol was being used, they found the animal might fall down but still be fully conscious, presumably in agony with a gaping hole in its head. 'We have seen the unpleasant effects of such ineffectual stunning where a semi-conscious animal has had to be dropped out of the box to be re-stunned,' they wrote. They also checked animals' skulls, to see just where the pistol had been aimed. 'In our view,' they reported, 'there were far too many cases where penetration had not been at or near the recommended position and also evidence of a considerable number of double shots [i.e. indicating that the first shot had missed its target].'

Bleeding to Death: Slaughtermen still generally believe that the animal's heart must be beating to drain its body of blood — thus all animals killed in slaughterhouses do, quite literally, bleed to death. During this, of course, they are supposed to be unconscious. The report questioned this assumption, and gave evidence to support the view that animals could and should be killed much quicker.

Slaughtermen who don't Know their Job: Slaughtermen are supposed to know how to stun animals (such as pigs) by holding electrical tongs onto their head and electrocuting them. For this, the tongs need to be applied for a *minimum* of seven seconds, otherwise the animal will simply not be unconscious. But they found a 'woeful ignorance of these requirements, which are frequently being disregarded.' They considered that the electricity was not applied properly in a high proportion of cases, and the slaughtermen were really only using the tongs to catch and immobilize animals. All this normally takes place in the full view of the other waiting animals, although the report did recommend that carcasses should not be 'dragged over other animals awaiting stunning nor should they be left in a position where they can be trampled by other animals.'

Unethical Tenderizing Techniques: Slaughtermen sometimes resort to artificial techniques aimed at making animal flesh more tender. These include giving the animal a special enzyme injection for a few minutes before it is slaughtered, and sending a low electrical current through the animal after it is stunned but before it is dead. Of the latter practice, they wrote: 'There are two areas for concern — (a) that an ineffectively stunned animal might be caused further suffering by use of this technique, and (b) that by delaying the sticking [i.e. bleeding to death] of an animal by up to sixty seconds while the process is being applied there is a greater risk that the effect of the initial stun might wear off and the animal therefore regain sensibility.' They considered the practice of giving an animal a tenderizing injection before it was slaughtered, which is not carried out with veterinary supervision, to be an unnecessary interference to the animal. Since incorrect dose or incorrect composition of the injection would cause the animal's death, one wonders what effect it might have on human consumers.

But many people disagree with that point of view. Research carried out at a New Zealand university found that calves were making attempts to get up off the floor five or six minutes after their throats had been cut. One Birmingham vet (Birmingham has four major slaughterhouses that are devoted to ritual killing), insists that it takes up to *twelve minutes* for the animal to lose consciousness. 'How would you feel about the same fate for your cat or dog?' he asks. 'There's no difference.'[6] Another vet explained to me that all animals (including humans) have several arteries supplying the brain, and not just the carotid ones that are slashed in ritual slaughter. He explained that another major artery, the vertebral one, ran close to the spinal column, and it would be quite impossible to sever this unless the whole head was cut off. Consequently, this artery goes on supplying blood to the brain even after the others have been cut, and so prolongs the animal's death.

In fact, most vets strongly dislike ritual slaughter. When the government's Farm Animal Welfare Committe working party prepared a report into the subject, they, too, concluded that it caused 'pain, suffering and distress,' and called for an end to slaughter without stunning within three years. But that's not likely.

Justifying the Unjustifiable

It seems difficult to understand how two of the world's great religions can sanction such a plainly barbaric practice. In fact, it is only strictly orthodox Jews and Muslims who insist on it, there being an increasing number of modern Jews and Muslims who are prepared to see the practice end.

Basically, there are two main reasons for the Jewish (*schechita* or *kosher*) and Islamic (*dhabbih* or *halal*) ways of slaughtering. First, the animal must be 'whole' if it is to be consumed by humans. This is taken to mean that it must not be sick or damaged in any way. It is therefore argued that pre-stunning, even if it occurs only a few seconds before death, is not acceptable since it results in a damaged animal. The second reason is to exsanguinate (bleed out) the animal, since consuming its blood is not permitted. But, in reality, it is *never* possible to drain all of the animal's blood from its body, as any vet can testify.

'Blood is unhealthy', says Dr. A. M. Katme, a representative of the Islamic Medical Association. 'It is full of toxins, urea, and organisms. The consumption of blood is forbidden for Muslims. It is arrogant for someone who is not a Muslim to presume that he can teach us the practice of our faith. God protect us from those who think that they know better than he.' [7]

But no animal can be fully drained of its blood and so, logically, Muslims who eat meat are actually contravening their own dietary laws. If they do not wish to consume blood, then, quite simply, they should not eat meat.

The Jewish method of cattle slaughter is particularly grosteque. Because cattle are large animals, they cannot be held down by slaughtermen. So instead, they are somehow driven into a small metal drum, that totally encloses them, leaving a small hole at the front for their head to stick out. Then the entire drum is rolled over, so that the cow is upside down, making it easier for the slaughterman to slash its neck. The chairman of the British Veterinary Association's Public Health Committee believe this causes the animal particular discomfort. 'It is likely to be very distressing,' he said. [5] The cow will usually thrash around so much in this upside down state that she will severely injure herself, and so technically render her a 'sick animal' and so be prohibited from being consumed by the orthodox. But this detail is often overlooked.

The Only Solution

When a senior diplomat at the Iranian embassy publicly slaughtered a sheep outside his house in Roehampton in September 1984, there was a large and angry public outcry. The diplomat was summoned to the British Foreign Office, and reprimanded for his behaviour. Unfortunately, this incident only serves to illustrate our double standards about the slaughter of animals. It seems that we are happy for it to go on, if it takes place in private. And we don't want to know what is done to these animals on our behalf, in our name. It's a clear case of out of sight, out of mind.

Realistically, there is little prospect of any meaningful reforms happening in the forseeable future. Any proposed changes will be heavily resisted or diluted by the meat industry if it threatens any of their profits. And the ritual slaughter question is just as likely to be blocked by interested parties.

It seems, therefore, that we as consumers have two possible choices. We could just accept the present state of affairs, and try to turn a blind eye to all the known barbarity and cruelty that routinely takes place on the factory farm and in the slaughterhouse. This is the option that most people follow at the moment.

Or we could refuse to be part of this brutal system by refusing to buy what it produces. Ultimately, this is the only course of action that will produce any real reform. Less consumer demand for cheap meat *at any price* will result in a reduction in the amount of animals that have to suffer for it. This, fundamentally, is what the meat industry is most frightened of. Because falling demand for meat plays havoc with their overheads, their high rates of turnover, and their highly geared profits.

Refusing to have an innocent animal's suffering and death on our conscience is a crucially important individual decision that re-asserts our own morality — our personal sense of what's right and what's wrong. But it actually goes even further than that. With each person who goes 'meat-free', so the economic pressure that market forces exert makes it more and more certain that one day soon the meat industry will, quite literally, become a dying business.

REFERENCES

1. The Guardian, 30 November 1984.
2. *Food in England*, Dorothy Hartley, Macdonald and Jane's, 1954.
3   Observed by Sarah Hicks and Jackie Bain.
4. 'Outrage', *Animal Aid*, November/December 1984 and September/October 1983.
5. 'What is Ritual Slaughter?' Mark Edmunds, *She*, July 1985.
6. *Birmingham Evening Mail*, 3 July 1985.
7. Letter to *The Guardian*, 20 August 1985.

11

What Every Body Needs

'More People are killed through the Stomach than by the Sword.'

— *Seneca*

For many (perhaps most) people, 'Nutrition' seems to be an impossible subject, very remote from them, and extremely difficult to understand. Personally, I attribute this to the very poor, or often non-existent, nutritional education many of us received while we were at school. Although things seem to be getting better now in some schools, there's still an awful long way to go.

Adults who never learnt to read when they were young face a very hard task when they try to learn the skill in later life. They find written English strange and foreign to them, full of complications and hard to master. Likewise, the vast majority of people go into adult life as nutritional 'illiterates', completely ignorant of the essential and basic knowledge they need to feed their bodies properly. It's really a scandal that this most important subject isn't included in *every* child's education.

Of course, there are lots of books around that can give you that basic information, if you're prepared to work your way through them. But most of us simply don't bother. There are other problems, too, that tend to discourage us from learning about our own nutrition. Some of them are:

- *Who do you believe?* Sometimes, it seems as if everyone's shouting conflicting advice at you. 'Eat high protein foods', 'Cut down on fats', 'Increase your polyunsaturated fats', 'Cut down on carbohydrates'. . . Frequently, this so-called advice comes from *very* interested parties, such as food manufacturers. And the bombardment starts early in life, with all the expensive, glossy 'information' packs that many manufacturers mail out to schools.

- *'Eating for Health by Albert Einstein'*. Many books are just too complicated, and so put off more people than they attract. With pages and pages of data, RDAs, and amino acids, and other technicalities, it's not surprising that you can end up thinking that nutrition is for geniuses only.

- *Grossed-Out on Diet Books*. Diet books are very big business, and it's been estimated that thirty per cent of all women try at least one diet in any year. Officially, thirty-two per cent of all women and thirty-nine per cent of all men in this country are classified as 'overweight', a horrifyingly high percentage. But the answer for these people *isn't* to buy one more fad book on dieting. First and foremost, it should be to learn the basics of good nutrition. Just cutting back on calories isn't going to help these people if they're not eating a balanced diet in the first place. If more people were to eat a *healthy* diet, there would be much less obesity around — and probably fewer diet books!

The Knowledge You Need

I don't want to bore you with endless facts and figures in this chapter, nor do I want to try to turn you into a nutrition freak. By cutting meat out of your diet, you have taken a very positive step forward towards establishing a good and healthy pattern of eating. But the job isn't over yet. To continue your progress, you should start to develop an awareness for the foods that go to make up a well-balanced intake, so that you *automatically* know when you and your family are eating well. What we're talking about here is dispelling *ignorance*. 'There is no sin but ignorance', said Christopher Marlowe in the 16th century. Ignorance of the basic facts breeds worry, which renders you vulnerable as a consumer to being misled or exploited. So first of all, let's answer some of the questions which seem to worry people most often.

'Give Me Back My Protein!'

Meat has very cleverly been identified with 'protein' in the mind of the public. Some people even think that meat is the *only* source of protein. So when you threaten to remove it from their diets, people tend to get upset. Once, when I was doing a phone-in on a radio station, a butcher phoned me to state in categoric terms that no-one could get enough protein without eating meat.

'That's very interesting,' I replied. 'Since you seem to know all about it, could you tell me what protein actually *is*?'

'Er,' he stumbled, 'Well I don't really know, but everyone needs it.'

'Well how much do we need?' I asked him.

'I don't know exactly,' he answered, 'but we all need lots.'

That was his total knowledge on the subject of protein, and I suspect that there are many others who are just as ignorant.

Protein is All Around Us

You can find protein in every living thing, plant and animal. Proteins are, quite simply, long collections of amino acids, which in turn are constructed from carbon, hydrogen, oxygen and nitrogen. Protein is naturally very plentiful. Next to water, it is the most plentiful substance in the human body. It helps build muscles, blood, skin, hair, nails, and our internal organs, as well as helping to create enzymes, antibodies and hormones. Also, the body can actually 'burn' protein if necessary to provide energy, at the rate of four calories of energy per gram of protein.

How much do you need? That depends on individual factors relating to you personally, such as your height, weight, sex and level of activity. Various organizations have produced recommendations, which have almost always been set at a very high level, partly to allow for a good 'safety margin'. There is a growing feeling that many such official bodies have set their recommendations much too high, and this has meant that authorities such as the U.N. Food and Agriculture Organisation have reduced their recommended levels of protein intake by as much as fifty per cent over the past fifteen years. The old idea that 'you can't get too much protein' is slowly dying, partly because excess protein intake is being associated with some degenerative diseases, such as osteoporosis (softening of the bones through calcium loss), obesity, and other curses of the Western way of living. Human milk is without doubt our most 'natural' food, and it is interesting that it contains a relatively small quantity of protein — less than thirty per cent of the protein that is found, for example, in cow's milk.

Using the Protein Calculator

To see what your own personal recommended daily protein intake is, use the Protein Calculator on page 207. This is based on figures that are suggested by Britain's Department of Health and Social Security.* First, find the category that applies to you (for example, a woman aged eighteen in a moderately active job would be in category U). Then read across to find your *minimum* protein requirement (in this case, 38 grams per day) and your *recommended* protein requirement (55 grams).

Now — just how easy is it to get this in your diet? Well, a selection of common meat-free foods is also given in the table. All you have to do is to follow the same row across the page until it is in the column corresponding to a food of your choice. For example, go to the column headed 'Pasta'. The notes at the end of the table will tell you that this is 100 per cent whole wheat spaghetti, and that one cup will provide 21 grams of protein. Now follow the 'Pasta' column down until you find your category (in our example, U). You will find a percentage figure that tells you what proportion of your Recommended Daily Allowance (R.D.A.) is supplied by 1 cup of

*Manual of Nutrition, Ministry of Agriculture, Fisheries and Food, HMSO 1979, used with permission.

pasta (in our example, one cup of whole wheat pasta provides 38.2 per cent of the Recommended Daily Allowance of protein for a woman aged eighteen with a moderately active lifestyle).

You may be surprised at just how easy it is to supply all the protein you need. And remember, this is a percentage of your *Recommended Daily Allowance* — not your *minimum* allowance. Here are some more foods that you should recognize as good suppliers of protein:

Grains	Legumes	Nuts
Whole Wheat	Soya Beans	Sunflower Seeds
Pasta	All Soya Products	Sesame Seeds
Bread	Kidney Beans	Tahini
Oats	Peas	Cashew Nuts
Rye	Lentils	Almonds
Rice (especially brown)	Bean Sprouts	Hazel Nuts
Barley	Peanuts	Coconuts
Millet	Chickpeas	Walnuts

In addition, dairy foods such as milk (skimmed preferably, to remove the excess fat), yogurt, eggs (free range), and cheese all contain useful quantities of protein.

Combining Foods to Maximize Protein

This is a useful tip for anyone who may be worried that they're eating a poor diet, and not getting enough protein. For the rest of us, it's just useful information.

It has been found that the maximum amount of protein is liberated from foodstuffs when they are *combined* together in the diet, and eaten at the same time. A very good combination is any grain product together with any legume — the two bring out each other's proteins very strongly. Another good combination is any legume with any nut. And either grains, legumes or nuts can be well combined with a dairy product. In fact, there are lots of dishes that naturally take advantage of this principle. Some of them are:

Macaroni and Cheese

Cereal and milk
Rice pudding
Pizza
Minestrone Soup
Peanut Butter Sandwich
Baked Potato and Cheese
Beans on Toast

And there are many, many more for you to devise yourself.

Calcium, the Body Builder

Everyone knows that calcium is necessary for healthy teeth and bones, but not everyone realizes that many people in this country could be at risk from calcium deficiency. A recent survey showed that many young teenagers are eating 'junk food' diets that are extremely inadequate sources of calcium. One scientist found that seventy-one per cent of young teenage girls would be calcium deficient, were it not for the calcium that has by law to be added to white bread. This is obviously a worrying state of affairs, particularly so when you consider that there have been recent attempts to 'relax' the law as far as adding calcium to white bread is concerned.

Meat is not a very good source of calcium, so cutting it out should not cause you any undue worry. However, *everyone*, whether they eat meat or not, should pay special attention to getting enough calcium in their diet.

Getting the Calcium You Need

Main sources of calcium are milk, cheese, bread and flour (if fortified) and green vegetables. Like other minerals and vitamins, calcium works with other dietary factors that increase or decrease the rate at which the body absorbs it. For example, some form of acid needs to be present for its proper assimilation, otherwise it cannot be dissolved into a water-soluble form and subsequently absorbed in the duodenum. Also, adequate amounts of Vitamin D are required to regulate the calcium balance in the blood. A good supply of Phosphorus, Vitamin A and Vitamin C are also needed.

The Recommended Daily Allowances for calcium are shown on page 210 in the Calcium Calculator. Ten good sources of calcium are also given, and the Nutrition-Checker system will allow you to work out the percentage of your R.D.A. for any food that you have information about (note — the British Dietetic Association does not recommend skim milk for children under 5 years of age, so no data is given. Dried milk is also unsuitable *unless* modified for infant use).

The Problem of Iron Deficiency

Lack of iron is the most common nutritional deficiency in this country. Once again, the fundamental cause is a poor basic diet, with an over-reliance on highly refined foods. In extreme form, iron deficiency will result in anaemia, whose symptoms may include pale skin, abnormal fatigue, constipation, brittle nails, and difficulty in breathing.

Nevertheless, the body manages its iron supply remarkably well. In normal circumstances, only about ten per cent of the iron in the diet will be absorbed, but in circumstances of deficiency the body will compensate by absorbing more. Also, the body will recycle its own supply of iron, generally only losing small amounts. Since over half of the body's supply of iron is normally found as haemoglobin in the blood, any loss of blood will deplete the body's store of iron.

Haemoglobin has the amazing quality of increasing the amount of oxygen that the blood can carry by *forty times*! Thus iron ensures that all our tissues get their essential supply of oxygen, and so helps us to increase our resistance to stress and infection. Iron is also needed to form myoglobin, which is only found in muscle tissue, and performs the same function as haemoglobin as it transports oxygen to the cells of our muscles as they exercise and contract.

Vitamins C and E help the body process iron in the diet, as do citric acid, calcium and sulphur-containing amino acids. Interestingly, the use of iron cooking utensils will provide a dramatic increase in the amount of iron found in foods cooked in them. It has been calculated that if spaghetti sauce is cooked for three hours in an iron pan, it will contain twenty-nine times as much iron as it would have contained if it had been cooked in glassware. However, since the dietary requirement for iron is basically a 'topping-up' function, it should be noted that it is possible to suffer from an overdose of iron. This may be caused by either a personal metabolic problem, or from excessive and prolonged dietary supplementation. As always, the best answer for normal individuals is to ensure that their diet naturally provides an optimum quantity of the element.

Where to Find Iron

About one quarter of the iron in the average meat-eater's diet is supplied by certain forms of meat, so cutting it out could potentially leave you with a twenty-five per cent shortfall — that is, if you don't eat anything else to replace your meat with! The main sources of iron in the diet are bread, flour and other cereal products, potatoes and green leafy vegetables. Some foods are extremely good sources of iron — such as prune juice (10mg in 256 grams), rolled oats (4.5mg in 100 grams), brewers yeast powder (4.3mg in 26 grams), dried apricots (4.1mg in 100 grams), raisins (3.5mg in 100 grams), plain chocolate (2.4mg in 100 grams), and broccoli (1.5mg in 100 grams). The Iron Calculator on page 212 shows you ten more good sources of iron. Note that when you use the Nutrition-Checker to analyse foods other than those listed, the weight of the food you want to eat should be in grams (as always), and the amount of iron should be in milligrams (mg).

A Cook's Tour of the World of Vitamins

Everyone knows that we all need vitamins, but what exactly are they? In this section we're going to have a whirlwind introduction to the wonderful world of vitamins, and, as before, focus particularly on those that may not be so plentiful in the average person's diet.

The importance of vitamins wasn't realized until the beginning of the twentieth century, when scientists began to find that tiny amounts of certain organic substances were essential to health. They called these organic substances 'vitamins', coming from the Latin word 'vita' (meaning life) coupled with the word 'amine', since they mistakenly believed that all vitamins contained amino acids (they don't).

Since they discovered that vitamins were either soluble in fat or in water, they also wrongly assumed that there were only two basic vitamins — and these they called Vitamin A (being fat soluble) and Vitamin B (being water soluble). We now know that there are well over twenty different vitamins, but they can still be divided into fat- or water- soluble types. Their basic work in the human body seems to be as the constituents of enzymes, which help to regulate our metabolism, converting fat and carbohydrate into energy, and helping us to make new tissue and bone.

Vitamins are called micro-nutrients, since the body only needs minute (but essential) quantities of them in the diet. Many people seem to have an almost magical faith in the power of vitamins, which the pill manufacturers are not slow to exploit. However, taking megadoses of synthetic vitamins is never preferable to getting a good supply of natural vitamins from a well-balanced diet. Vitamins work in complex and inter-related ways in the human body — and they never work alone. A synthetic vitamin pill can never replicate the delicate relationship that exists between different vitamins in nature, and relying on such pills may actually be harmful. Large doses of fat-soluble vitamins (such as A, D, E and K) will tend to accumulate in the body and may eventually prove toxic. Water soluble vitamins are much less toxic in large doses, but still may produce symptoms of overdose. As always, it's a question of getting the balance right!

Vitamin A

Vitamin A (retinol) is formed in the healthy human body from carotene, which is a substance that gives a yellow or orange colour to plants. Fruits or vegetables of these colours are therefore likely to be good vitamin A sources. Diabetics have problems in converting carotene into vitamin A, and should therefore be careful to ensure that they are not retinol deficient. Vitamin A is stored in our livers, and its functions include helping new cells to grow, as well as the more well-known one of aiding night vision (this aspect of vitamin A became publicised in World War Two, when the British Government tried to conceal their development of radar by attributing the success of their bombing missions over Germany to the high doses of vitamin A that the crews were taking). It has also been used externally to treat cases of acne, impetigo, boils, carbuncles, ulcers, and to promote the healing of wounds.

Too much vitamin A will cause toxic symptoms, which may include headaches, sickness, irritability, and (in severe cases) growth retardation in children. On the other hand, a deficiency of Vitamin A in the diet will eventually cause a general weakening and increased susceptibility to many kinds of infection — probably including cancers. It is thought that this happens when our cell walls (which vitamin A gives strength and protection to) become more susceptible to invading bacteria. In some countries, vitamin A deficiency can be a serious problem. It has been estimated that as many as 80,000 children go blind every year due to lack of vitamin A, and about half of them will die as a direct result.

Cooked vegetables are actually higher in usable vitamin A than raw ones, because the plant cell membranes are destroyed during cooking, thus making more carotene available for our bodies to convert to vitamin A proper (retinol). However, high-temperature cooking will tend to destroy or degrade it.

Measuring the amount of vitamin A in foods can be somewhat complicated, since some sort of allowance has to be made for the carotene-retinol conversion process carried out by the body. The Recommended Daily Allowances give a *retinol-equivalent* figure for vitamin A in micrograms. This measures the final amount of vitamin A that ends up in our bodies, coming from whatever source. However, sometimes the amount of vitamin A in foods is given in International Units (I.U.), and then the following conversion will have to be undertaken to arrive at a *retinol equivalent* figure:

- For *Plant Food Sources*: devide the amount of B-carotene measured in I.U.s by ten to calculate the retinol equivalent.
- For *Animal Food Sources*: multiply the amount of retinol measured in I.U.s by 0.3 to calculate the retinol equivalent.
- Where vitamin A is measured in micrograms of B-carotene, this figure should be divided by six to calculate the retinol equivalent (except for milk, when it should be divided by two).

Vitamin A is not found in all foods by any means, so here is a list of some of the better sources, together with the amount of vitamin A they contain, stated as retinol equivalents. The quantities of each food have been standardized to 100 grams, to enable a quick comparison to be made:

Margarine (fortified)	900
Mustard Greens (cooked)	820
Cress (cooked)	770
Watercress	500
Endive (raw)	330
Pimentos (tinned)	230
Mela (ogen/canteloupe)	175
Egg	140
Tomatoes	100
Peaches	83
Peas (raw)	64
Cabbage	50
Green Pepper (raw)	43

Finally, one interesting source of Vitamin A is the spice paprika, which contains 127 micrograms (retinol equivalent) in just one teaspoonful!

The B Group Vitamins

Not long ago, I was asked by the BBC to appear on the Six O'Clock

News to explain the reasons underlying the phenomenal increase in the number of people who don't eat meat. To balance the programme, they had also invited the head of the Meat Promotion Executive (the man who is paid to try to sell meat to you and me). After I had told the newscaster why I believed more and more people were going meat-free, the meat man had his say. Amongst other things, he said that the meat producers had been silent for far too long (some joke, considering the size of their advertising budgets), and he intimated that they now intended to fight this insidiously rising tide of non-meat eating. Then, as he continued talking about health and protein, I began to understand the sort of tactics they were going to use. One remark, in particular, stuck in my head. 'Meat is a vital source of B vitamins,' he said.

'So that's it,' I thought to myself. 'They can't sell it to us by making it desirable, so they're going to frighten us by making us believe we can't live healthily without it.'

Unfortunately, the item finished at that point, so I didn't have the opportunity to tell the meat man (and seven million viewers) that he was talking rubbish. But, of course, he was. Meat is *not* a 'vital' source of B vitamins. In fact, it's not a 'vital' source of anything. There is no nutrient contained in meat that cannot be obtained from other sources.

The B group vitamins, however, *are* vital to human well-being, and everyone ought, for their own sakes, to know what they are and where to find them. This sort of knowledge gives you power — the power to refuse to be exploited or manipulated by commercial interests when they try to sell you their products by telling 'little white lies'.

So what are the B group vitamins? Chemically, they are all rather different, but they do have certain things in common. They are all soluble in water and so pass through the body quite quickly (this means we need a regular source of them in our diet). They are produced from bacteria, yeasts and moulds, and so tend to naturally occur together in nature. Most of them can therefore be found in yeast products (brewer's yeast, or yeast extracts), and wholegrain cereals are another good source.

We need B group vitamins to help us convert the carbohydrate in our diet into usable energy, and they also help the nervous system to function properly. We need more B vitamins during times of infection, stress or high activity, and heavy alcohol and coffee drinkers also need a higher than normal intake. A typically highly-processed 'junk food' diet does not contain an adequate level of these vitamins, and, if this applies to you, this is one more good reason to take a greater interest in your food habits! A deficiency of these vitamins may lead to irritability, depression, and in extreme cases even suicide. Grey or falling hair, insomnia, poor appetite and constipation are more signs of possible deficiency.

Vitamin B_1 (*Thiamin*) is fairly plentifully supplied in many natural food sources. The Recommended Daily Allowances (R.D.A) for Thiamin range from 0.3mg (for infants under 1 year) to 1.4mg (for very active males). As a rule, the more active you are, the more thiamin you need, and the more carbohydrate you take in (this includes alcohol) the more thiamin you need. Most of this can be supplied by a single tablespoonful (8 grams) of brewer's yeast, which contains 1.2mg of thiamin. Other good sources include millet (0.85mg in half a cup, dry), peas (0.45mg in one cup, cooked), broccoli (0.48mg in 3 stalks, cooked), wheat germ (1.6mg in one cup), and sunflower seeds (1.42mg in half a cup). It is not known whether there are any toxic effects in cases of overdose.

Vitamin B_2 (*Riboflavin*) is also quite widely distributed in foods, although many foods contain very small amounts. Lack of riboflavin is believed to be one of the most common vitamin deficiencies in the West. For this reason, we show on page 000 a complete Riboflavin Calculator, which will enable you to check your own intake. About a third of the average intake of riboflavin in this country is provided by milk, and since riboflavin can be destroyed by ultra-violet light, milk should not be left exposed to sunlight. Deficiency of riboflavin is believed to lead to a lack of stamina and to retard human growth, and may result in certain visual problems, including cataracts. Some good sources are given in the Calculator.

Vitamin B_6 (*Pyridoxine*) in the absence of official D.H.S.S. recommendations for the R.D.A. of this vitamin, it is suggested that the Canadian Dietary Standard be followed, which is given on page 220.

Pyridoxine is found in whole grains and brewer's yeast. Some good sources are: avocado (0.84g in one average); skim milk (0.1mg in one cup); yeast extract (0.24mg in one tablespoon); wheat germ (1.1mg in one cup, toasted); orange juice (1mg in one unsweetened cup); raisins (0.4 in one cup); roasted peanuts (0.5mg in one cup); sunflower seeds (1.8mg in one cup); walnuts (0.73mg in one cup); cauliflower (0.22mg in one cup, cooked or raw); tomato juice (0.37mg in one cup); broccoli (0.89mg in 3 stalks raw); and banana (0.61mg in one average).

Vitamin B_{12} is the only B vitamin that does not occur in plants (it does occur in some fermented plant foods, since it is produced by a micro-organism, like a mould). The suggested daily intake is 3 micrograms, and 4 micrograms for pregnant or lactating women. This can be easily supplied as follows: skim milk (1mcg in one cup); soya milk (4mcg in one cup of fortified soya milk); cheddar (1.12mcg in 4 ounces); cottage cheese (2.4mcg in one cup); yeast extract (usually enough for an adult's R.D.A., but amount may vary, check the label); and most health food shops will also sell other products that have vitamin B_{12} in them too.

Folic Acid is particularly abundant in green leafy vegetables (the name comes from 'foliage'), but is not commonly found in meat or meat products. In addition, it is easily destroyed by cooking *unless* it is protected by a naturally acidic environment, such as ascorbic acid (vitamin C). Cooking and re-heating food may destroy virtually all the folic acid it contains, so this is an excellent reason to ensure that your diet always contains a good quantity of *fresh* green leafy vegetables, and to shun over-processed, stale, junk food. A suggested intake is 400 micrograms for adults, 800 micrograms in pregnancy and 600 during lactation. Deficiency of this vitamin will result in poor growth, anaemia, susceptibility to infection, and recent research has associated lack of folic acid with certain forms of mental illness. It has been used to treat patients suffering from atherosclerosis, stomach ulcers, menstrual problems, and even grey hair!

Here are some good sources: brewer's yeast (192mcg in one tablespoonful); yeast extract (240mcg in one tablespoonful); raw beetroot (126mcg in 1 cup, try it grated in a salad, delicious!); cooked spinach (164mcg in 1 cup); wheat germ (420mcg in 1 cup, toasted); orange juice (136mcg in one cup); almonds (136mcg in one cup); roasted peanuts (153mcg in one cup); black eye beans (168mcg in one cup, cooked) and broccoli (219mcg in 3 pieces, cooked).

Nicotinic Acid is part of the B group that occurs in several forms — including niacin, nicotinamide, and niacinamide. Once again, it is easy to obtain, being available both in a direct dietary form and also being synthesized internally by the body from the amino acid tryptophan (found in nuts, dairy products and pulses). Some good sources are: nori (10mg in 100 grams), brewers yeast powder (9.4mg in 25 grams), barley (dry, 3.7mg in 100 grams), and dried apricots (3.3mg in 100 grams). The suggested intake of nicotinic acid (or nicotinic acid equivalent), as recommended by the D.H.S.S., is shown below. Since individual take-up and conversion of nicotinic acid can vary considerably from person to person, these figures are set well above the minimum amount needed by most bodies.

	Age	Nicotinic Acid (mg)
Children	Under 1 year	5
	1 year	7
	2 years	8
	3-4 years	9
	5-6 years	10
	7-8 years	11
Males	9-11 years	14
	12-14 years	16
	15-17 years	19
sedentary	18-34 years	18
mod. active	18-34 years	18
very active	18-34 years	18
sedentary	35-64 years	18
mod. active	35-64 years	18

Age		Nicotinic Acid (mg)
very active	35-64 years	18
	75 & over	15
Pregnant		18
Lactating		21

Since the amino acid tryptophan is converted into nicotinic acid by the body at the rate of 60mg tryptophan to 1mg nicotinic acid, and since it is not easy to determine how much tryptophan is present in foods, no Nutrition-Checker information is given for this vitamin. However, it is quite easy to obtain a good supply of nicotinic acid in the diet, and the following list gives some foods that have a plentiful supply of it:

Food	Measure	Nicotinic Acid Equivalent (mg)
Tofu	4 ounces (120 grams)	15.6
Soya Beans	half cup dry	11.5
Avocado	one average	8
Cheddar	4 ounces (120 grams)	7.44
Lentils	half cup dry	5.3
Chickpeas	half cup dry	4.8
Yeast Extract	one tablespoon	4.4
Peas	4 ounces (120 grams)	3.6
Peanut Butter	one tablespoon	3.4
Mango	one medium	3
Mushrooms	3 large raw	3
Millet	quarter cup dry	2.5
Potatoes	4 ounces (120 grams)	2.04
Sunflower Seeds	2 tablespoons	2
Banana	one large	1.4

*From data in *Laurel's Kitchen*, L. Robertson, C. Flinders, B. Godfrey, (Routledge and Kegan Paul).

Pantothenic Acid is another B group vitamin that works closely with the others to metabolize fat and carbohydrate into energy that the body can use. It is very widely found in natural foods (although processing and freezing will destory it) and the Ministry of Agriculture Fisheries and Food comment in their *Manual of Nutrition*: 'Dietary deficiencies of this vitamin are unlikely in man because it is so widespread in food.' A good supply of the other B group vitamins will ensure that you get enough Pantothenic Acid.

Vitamin C

Vitamin C has suffered from a lot of hype for its alleged 'miracle' properties, but, notwithstanding all that, it's still quite an incredible vitamin. Humans are almost alone (apart from the great apes and some guinea pigs) in our dietary need for it — most other animals can synthesize it in their own bodies but, since we can't, we need to take in a regular supply of it in our diet. This isn't always easy. A diet that contains a large proportion of meat, oils, tea, coffee, alcohol, pastry and other refined carbohydrate foods (and any processed foods) may well be vitamin C deficient. In other words, a typical meat-oriented, fast food diet. As the Ministry of Agriculture Fisheries and Food say: 'this vitamin remains one of the few nutrients in which the British diet can be deficient.'

What happens when you suffer from a lack of vitamin C? Well eventually, you contract scurvy and die (scurvy was the curse of the early long-distance sailors who couldn't obtain fresh fruit and vegetables). But long before that, you will begin to suffer from sub-scurvy symptoms. The onset of these symptoms is quite quick once your diet becomes vitamin C deficient. They include: bleeding from the gums and from small blood vessels (causing tiny red dots of blood to be visible under the skin), poor stamina and general debility, shortness of breath, easy bruising, nosebleeds, anaemia, slow healing of wounds and a marked decrease in your resistance to infections. Since blood clots may form at the point where your capillary wall has ruptured, it is quite likely that vitamin C deficiency may predispose people to heart attacks and strokes.

The function of vitamin C in the human body is basically to promote the formation of connective tissue, and so it plays an important role in the body's continuing regeneration of itself, as well as in healing wounds. It helps to fight bacterial infection and may reduce the effect of certain allergies on the human body. It's needed by the bones and teeth to keep them healthy and strong, and also helps metabolize certain proteins. It has also been found to protect other vitamins against destruction in the body before they can be fully utilized. These are just some of the functions that vitamin C fulfills — as you can see, it's a pretty useful substance.

The suggested intake of vitamin C ranges from 15mg a day for children under one year, to 60mg a day for pregnant or lactating women. The average R.D.A. is about 30mg a day. Don't rely on cooked food to give you this. In fact, you can't even rely on *raw* food, if it's several days old, because vitamin C decays rapidly, and is sensitive to light and heat. Cooking vegetables in copper pans will also destroy vitamin C. For these reasons, and because the amount of vitamin C in foods can very widely, we can't really give Nutrition-Checker data for this vitamin, but we can tell you where you're likely to find it in the sort of amounts that you need.

As vitamin C is generally well-preserved in acid environments, citrus fruits are usually a good source. One cup of fresh orange juice may give you as much as 120mg, which is enough to satisfy anyone's R.D.A. Other good sources are red and green peppers, bean sprouts (sprout them yourself to ensure perfect freshness, it's easy and they're much more tasty than supermarket ones), potatoes, spinach (one cup cooked will give you about 50mg), cabbage, broccoli and brussels sprouts.

Some people have indulged in massive doses of vitamin C, and report that it can treat, among other things, the common cold, hepatitis, herpes simplex, and drug addiction. Some symptoms are associated with continual over-dose, such as skin rashes, loose bowels, and a burning sensation during urination, but these are associated with very considerable intakes, up to 15,000mg per day. There seems to be little point in taking such massive doses of vitamin C, since what the body cannot use is immediately discharged into the urine. It would be more sensible to take smaller, more frequent doses that the body can more easily process — preferably, by eating a good fresh diet.

Smoking will deplete the body of vitamin C, by anything up to one-third of the total amount present. Other kinds of stress will also result in depletion, and this should be taken account of in the diet. Also, our need for vitamin C may increase with age, since the body has a greater need to regenerate its collagen. A dirty environment — such as the urban pollution that most of us now have to contend with — may also increase our need for this vitamin.

Vitamin D

This has been called the 'Sunshine Vitamin', because (even in our grey climate) that is precisely where most of us get it from. The sun's rays act on a fat contained in our skin, and convert it into vitamin D. This is a pretty efficient process and, perhaps surprisingly, most people get enough vitamin D this way.

Vitamin D is dissolved in fat, rather than water, and so the body finds it less easy to flush any excess out of the system. Consequently, in order to prevent a toxic dose, vitamin D dietary supplementation should only take place under medical supervision when it is known that a deficiency exists, or for pregnant or lactating women.

Some food sources of vitamin D include: skim milk (if specially fortified), whole milk, egg yolk, butter, seafood and cream. Margarine is also fortified with it. It helps to prevent rickets, and generally helps in teeth and bone growth and development.

Vitamin E

This vitamin, once again, is not found to much extent in meat or meat products. The main sources are cereals, eggs, and vegetable oils — indeed, such vitamin E as exists in meat is derived, by the animal, from a plant source.

There are several different types of vitamin E, all called tocopherols. They are fat soluble, and act essentially as preservatives or anti-oxidants. Food processing will remove much of the vitamin E it contains, so cold-pressed vegetable oils are to be preferred on this account (yes, they may be more expensive, but they're worth it, and the higher price may discourage you from using too much). A meat-orientated diet that is high in saturated fat and low in vitamin

E, may lead to the formation of various harmful products of fat decomposition in the body.

On the other hand, there should be no need in a well-balanced meat-free diet to worry about vitamin E deficiency. Some naturally good sources are: wheat germ, sunflower oil, soya oil, and most nuts and seeds.

A Note About Mothers and Babies

The best possible preparation for pregnancy and childbirth is a good balanced diet *before* you get pregnant. You ought to pay particular attention to getting sufficient protein, iron, calcium, vitamin D and B group vitamins, as your body's requirement for these will increase considerably during pregnancy. You should be able to find a sympathetic, modern physician who understands meat-free nutrition quite easily. Also, it's another good opportunity to learn something more about your own body and its requirements, so try to make time to do some reading, you'll find it very worthwhile. There are several books that specialize in meatless nutrition for mothers and babies, a particularly useful one being *The Vegetarian Baby* by Sharon Yntema (published by Thorsons).

For the first few months your baby will need little more than mother's milk (during which time your own nutritional needs will change somewhat, your body requiring slightly less protein, but more vitamin A, vitamin C, B group, iodine and zinc). At about six months the baby will be able to eat some solids, and by nine months food such as grains, beans, bread, fruit or vegetables will be taken if they are well softened and/or ground first. Remember that all beans and pulses *must* be well cooked and thoroughly boiled, it is dangerous just to simmer them or soften them in a slow cooker. This is how Sharon Yntema suggests various foods may be introduced into your baby's diet, and at what stage:

4-5 months:
Introduce: ripe banana, avocado, pear, sweet potatoes, yogurt. All food should be finely mashed or puréed'.
Amounts: single food per meal, one meal a day (breast feeding still main source of food).

5-6½ months:
Introduce: grains (rice, barley, millet, oatmeal), more vegetables (peas, butter beans, green beans), more fruits and fruit juices. All food should be puréed or fork-mashed.
Amounts: one or two foods at a meal, two meals a day, juice for a snack once a day (breast feeding still substantial).

6½-8 months:
Introduce: egg yolks, stronger flavoured vegetables such as cabbage, spinach, broccoli, kale. Main meal should be in puréed form. Finger foods should be soft. Pre-soaked dried fruits and bread pieces are good finger food.
Amounts: two to three meals a day or two meals plus finger foods snack (breast feeding at least twice a day).

8-9 months
Introduce: legumes, tofu, nut and seed pastes, cheese, bulgur, any other vegetables, fruits or grains that have not previously been introduced. Meals can be in less puréed form, but there should be no hard or large chunks. Finger foods can be chunkier.
Amounts: three meals a day plus finger food snacks (breast feeding twice a day).

New food should be introduced slowly, one thing at a time so that your baby can get used to new flavours and food textures. Some things will be popular, some won't — and your baby will exercise his or her preferences just like anyone else! You will find certain equipment, such as a food processor or liquidizer very useful for grinding and milling, and also for making puréed fruits and vegetables (canned baby food is expensive and it's better to make your own if you're able).

Bringing a new life into the world is one of the most meaningful experiences that humans can have. Generations of people have proved for themselves that a baby can be raised happily and healthily (some would say *more* healthily) without including meat from animals in its diet. Even the very thought of feeding a young life on dead flesh is repugnant to many people. So go ahead — learn everything you can, and be confident that you really are doing the right thing!

12

The Baby that Eats Five People

> The solution to the problems of developing countries must lie in international finance. The proposition that boycotting or significantly reducing meat consumption will affect this process is not only an unnecessary distraction from important issues, it can be positively harmful through its effect on commodity prices.[1]

Bland, reassuring words. Words uttered by the director of planning and development of the Meat and Livestock Commission — the people whose job it is to ensure that we carry on eating meat. How nice to know that 'international finance' can solve the problems of a hungry world, a world in which *five hundred million* people go hungry every day. A world in which *four hundred thousand* children die every day from hunger and hunger-related diseases.[2] And it can all be solved by 'international finance'.

But 'international finance' *hasn't* solved these problems. 'International finance' probably doesn't give a damn. And nor does the meat industry.

Feeding the Rich, Starving the Poor

Many people are so hideously misinformed about the world food situation that they actually believe that the world doesn't have the resources to feed everyone. 'There's not enough land,' they say.

This is rubbish. 'There *is* enough land to grow food,' says the charity Oxfam. 'Who it feeds, what it is used for and what it grows — those are the problems.' Oxfam cites one example of the misuses of arable land in Brazil like this: 'In Brazil huge cattle ranches take up some of the most fertile soil in the whole country, yet sixty per cent of Brazilians are malnourished.'

This is a familiar pattern in many developing countries, who are forced to squander their own resources in order to produce cheap beef for the affluent West to consume. Since much of this imported meat goes to make cheap meat products, such as hamburgers, the process has been called 'hamburgerization'. The net result of today's 'hamburgerization' is not so very far removed from Jonathan Swift's bitterly satirical proposal in the eighteenth century that the rich should eat the babies of the poor, and so solve the world food problem once and for all. And yet 'hamburgerization' is real, and is going on all the time, in the name of the ever-hungry meat consumer of the West.

The poor, the malnourished, and the starving aren't the only casualties of this immoral business. The massive forests of Central America are falling under the meat-baron's axe — more than sixty per cent of the forests have disappeared in the last thirty years. After all, a beef steer needs a lot of room to graze.

And the birds are dying, too. As their habitat diminishes, their numbers are falling — not a slow and gentle decline, but a sharp and brutal decimation. Scientists at the Smithsonian Institute say that the forest songbirds are declining at between one and four per cent *every year.* Since these birds migrate to the North American agricultural heartland, scientists believe that their drastic decrease will mean a sharp increase in the number of crop pests that the birds used to keep under control. Well, at least it's good news for the pesticide manufacturers.[3] The picture in other countries is just as bad. In Australia, for example, 300,000 wild horses are being slaughtered at the command of American beef buyers, who believe that the horses may pass on disease to the beef cattle. The mass slaughter is so large that the beef barons charter helicopters and use them as gunships, spraying the horses with bullets from the air. In Britain, our own Ministry of Agriculture has pursued an extermination policy against badgers for much the same reasons, despite mounting scientific evidence that our badgers are not implicated in the spread of disease to cattle.

But what can you and I actually *do* about this act of rape, being perpetrated in the name of the affluent Western consumer? If we listen to the meat industry, there is nothing we can do. We are powerless. We should leave the problem of world hunger to 'international finance' to sort out. And while we're waiting, we can help ourselves to another hamburger.

But the meat industry is wrong — we *can* make things change, if we want to. In reality, none of us is powerless. As consumers, we are actually part of one of the most powerful pressure groups on the face of this planet, if we only realised it. But in order to make things change for the better, we first need to know the full truth. And there's one very important fact that the meat industry will *never* tell us . . .

Meat Production is an Obscene Waste of Human Food

The fact is stark and simple. Meat as a food can never — *will* never — feed the world. Economically, it just can't be done. And the more meat *we* eat, the less food there is available for other people.

A meat animal is nothing more or less than a machine — a machine that the industry uses to convert vegetable protein into animal protein. As a machine, it is deplorably inefficient. For every kilo of meat protein that is produced as a steak, *twenty kilos* of vegetable protein have to be put into it. Twenty kilos that *could* have gone to make vital human food. Twenty kilos that *might* have prevented someone, somewhere from starving to death. It is a disgraceful, obscene waste of food. The next chart shows you just what inefficient 'machines' food animals are:[4]

As you can see, beef animals are the most wasteful converters of foodstuff, only managing to convert a miserly six per cent of the vegetable protein they are fed into meat protein. This is the reason behind the desperate use of hormones in animal rearing — it's an attempt by the farmer to improve on the process that at

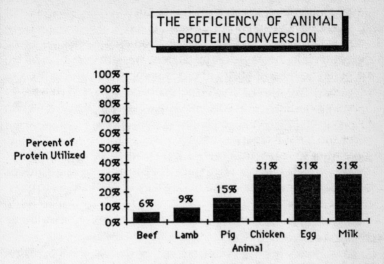

least one beef producer has described as 'notoriously inefficient'. So where does the other ninety-four per cent of food input actually go? 'It's wasted, of course. Just disposing of all that excrement causes considerable pollution problems. Even the most efficiently produced animal foods (chickens, eggs, milk) only use thirty-one per cent of the protein from their feedstuff, wasting the remaining two thirds.

The Meat Industry Can't Break the Laws of Nature — But it Can Hide the Consequences

This system of food production is so outrageously inefficient, because the meat producers are trying (and inevitably failing) to break one of the most fundamental laws of nature. This is the law that explains, amongst other things, why large, fierce animals are comparatively rare, but smaller, vegetable-feeding ones are much more numerous.

In the wild, food chains exist whereby one 'level' of the chain consumes something on a lower level of the chain. At the bottom of the chain, there are lots and lots of animals feeding on a profusion of plentiful foodstuff (for example, rabbits feeding on grass). At the top of the chain, there are just a few fierce animals who feed on the lower levels (foxes feeding on rabbits). Thus, the foxes are indirectly eating the lowest level of the chain — grass.

If things get out of balance, and the fox population suddenly expands, there won't be enough rabbits to go round. So the foxes just starve until things get back into balance again.

By rights, therefore, if humans were designed to be predominantly carnivores, and exist on flesh foods, there would be relatively few of us, living at a good distance from each other. It's quite obvious, however, that we're *not* like that. Humans are not carnivorous creatures, and there are far too many of us to live at such a perilously high position in the food chain. But that's where the meat industry ignores nature. The consequence of this perversion of nature is continual enforced starvation for hundreds of millions of our fellow humans. However, most of us don't realize that the meat industry is playing this grotesque game with nature.

Need or Greed? It's Your Choice

Let's look at this problem from another point of view. If you had an acre of average quality land, and wanted to get the maximum amount of protein that you could use for human consumption out of it, what would you choose to do with it. The next graph gives you a clue.[5]

That's right — vegetable sources of protein will give you *many* times more protein than even the best animal source (milk). And beef production is the worst possible use that you could put your land to, being nearly twenty times less productive of usable protein than soya beans. So you'd be stupid to use your land for beef, wouldn't you? Stupid, that is, unless you were being coerced by economic pressure to produce beef. Which is precisely what happens. In Mexico, for example, Oxfam estimate that eighty per cent of the children in rural areas are under-nourished, and yet the livestock are fed more grain than the *whole population eats*. What happens to the livestock? They are exported, of course, to satisfy

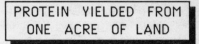

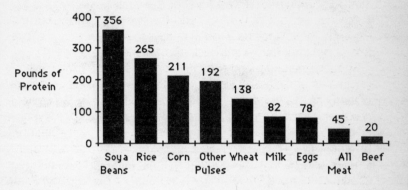

PROTEIN YIELDED FROM ONE ACRE OF LAND

Foodstuff

the developed nations' craving for cheap hamburgers. If economic pressure can bring about this crazy state of affairs, it follows that we, the consumers (who are the ultimate source of *all* economic demand) — *can* influence the way that our world goes about producing its food.

And while you're chewing that over, here are some more facts that you ought to know:

- The average meat-eating Westerner munches his way through one ton (about a thousand kilograms) of grain every year.[6] Ninety-three per cent of this is eaten indirectly, in the form of meat and meat products. On the other hand, the average Indian consumes 180 kilograms of grain every year — the vast majority of it efficiently eaten as direct cereal products.
- Economists have calculated that if the Western world was to cut its meat consumption by just fifty per cent, each person doing so would release enough grain to keep two more people alive, who would otherwise starve.[7]
- The meat industry has even begun to export this particular brand of economic lunacy to many third world countries, and British

companies (no doubt using 'foreign aid' funding) have recently sold complete intensive livestock systems to Zambia, Zimbabwe, Kenya, Cameroon, Sudan, Nigeria, and Bangladesh. Many of these countries don't even have enough grain to feed their *people*. But our Western lifestyle has been sold so seductively to their governments, who are eager to imitate their affluent neighbours, that the harsh economic realities don't appear to have been taken into consideration.[8]

- Ninety-five per cent of the soya bean harvest — which is one of the greatest sources of protein in the world — is fed straight to animals. Only 1.5 per cent of the crop is used directly by humans. This criminal wastage is almost impossible to comprehend.

- It is not just in economic terms that the meat industry is trying to fiddle the books. In terms of energy use, animal food production is also unbelievably inefficient. Let's compare the energy used in modern oat or potato production with that used in beef production.[9] For every one calorie of fossil fuel expended, oats produce 2.47 food calories, and potatoes produce 2.18 calories. But beef only returns 0.03 of a calorie — it actually *loses* ninety-seven per cent of the energy that's put in. How long can we go on wasting our resources like this?

These are some of the basic facts that you should know — that everyone who chooses to eat meat should know.

The truth is uncomfortable for us, and is very easy to ignore. Whenever we see those haunting, horrific images of starvation on television, it is tempting to blame it all on politics, on corrupt governments, or ignorant farmers, or on 'international finance'. But that is just running away from the problem.

The inescapable reality is this. That every steak a Westerner consumes could have provided enough food for *five people* who don't eat meat. That every baby who is brought up in our Western world to eat meat will consume *five times* as much of the planet's food resources as a child who does not eat meat.

It's our decision.

REFERENCES

1. *Super Marketing*, December 1985.
2. Oxfam figures.
3. 'How the song birds choked on fast food', Myers, N., *Guardian*, 6 December 1984.
4. From data in 'Biological Ceilings and Economic Efficiencies for the Production of Animal Protein A.D.2000', Wilson, P. N., *Chemistry and Industry*, 6 July 1968.
5. U.S.D.A. per-acre yield statistics 1971-74, WHO/FAO/UNICE Protein Advisory Group Bulletin No. 6, 1971.
6. *Animal Liberation*, Peter Singer, Thorsons.
7. Ibid, and New York Times, 25 October 1974.
8. 'Why do chickens cross the Globe?' Gold, M., *Guardian*, 28 December 1984.
9. A *Vegetarian Sourcebook*, Akers, K., G. P. Putnam's Sons, New York.

13

Changes

'Let the great world spin for ever
down the ringing grooves of change.'

— Tennyson, *Locksley Hall*

The very essence of human life is surely our amazing ability to grow, to develop, and to create something more out of ourselves than empirical evidence would suggest was possible. But we only grow as human beings in direct proportion to our willingness to accept change. If death can be defined as the cessation of conscious control of change, then life has to be precisely the opposite — a continual manifestation of this near-miraculous human talent to control and change our individual and collective destinies.

Judged by this standard, not many people could be said to be truly 'alive' at the moment. And yet this ability is one of our fundamental birthrights — perhaps *the* essential quality that distinguishes us from other animals. As a species, we assumed control of our destiny two million years ago, when our ancestors rose to the challenge presented to them by an increasingly hostile environment. Their choice was stark — evolve, or perish. Now, we face the same decision again.

Change has never been easy for Homo *sapiens*, and we have always had to be prodded quite hard by nature (or circumstances, if you prefer), before we would do very much about it. Well, the prods are getting much, much sharper now. We are faced with many grave and insistent problems, which we ignore only at our most extreme peril. Our species is being ravaged by degenerative diseases on a scale that we have never seen before. Many of our fellow beings are dying because some of our number choose to consume far more of our earth's food resources than their need entitles them to. And the way we treat the creatures that share this planet with us reveals that many of us are still immature enough to believe that all other lifeforms are basically second-class, and only matter in as much as they amuse or make themselves useful to us.

It's Time to Decide

Our world is fast approaching crisis point. Each of us has to decide where we stand — to choose between change, or no-change. For all practical purposes, it's a decision between life and death/or, in more dramatic terms, between good and evil. The battle lines have never before been so clearly drawn, nor so unequally balanced. On the side of no-change, are all the tyrants, despots, power-hungry, selfish and short-sighted people of the world, who will resist any challenge to their dominion. These people (and there are many of them) share a common unspoken philosophy — they believe that humans have no obligations to each other, nor to their fellow creatures, nor to the planet as a whole. They believe that Might is Right, and that the strongest has license to exploit the weakest. This is how one of their number presents their case:

'The beast of prey is the highest form of active life,' wrote the Nazi philosopher Oswald Spengler in 1931. 'It represents a mode of living which requires the extreme degree of the necessity of fighting, conquering, annihilating, self-assertion. The human race ranks highly because it belongs to the class of beasts of prey. Therefore we find in man the tactics of life proper to a bold, cunning beast of prey. He lives engaged in aggression, killing, annihilation. He wants to be master in as much as he exists.'

The Older Wisdom

Even the most optimistic of us have to admit that Spengler's doctrine of evil is a pervasive force that shapes our society to a large extent at the moment. Nevertheless, there is an older, universal wisdom which suggests that things might not have to be this way. . .

The Cherokee Indians have a tribal myth that says that humans once lived in perfect harmony with all their fellow creatures and plants, and all of them could speak to each other. In China, the Taoist Chuang Tsu wrote in the fourth century B.C. of a past 'age of virtue' when all humankind lived a common co-operative life with the birds and the beasts. And in Greece, the philosopher Empedocles wrote of a 'golden age, an age of love' when 'no altar was wet with the shameful slaughter of bulls,' and he maintained that the primal sin was man's slaughter of animals.

Many cultures, in fact, have ancient myths that speak of an early period (usually the earliest) of their existence, and tell how, through folly or evil, humankind fell from a state of grace and equality with all creatures and became a tyrant and despot. The Old Testament tells us that the world that God creates is, initially, perfect. It is quite clear that in this perfect state, it is not intended for humans to eat the flesh of other creatures. God says:

'Behold I have given you every herb yielding seed, which is upon the face of the earth, and every tree, in which is the fruit of a tree yielding seed; to you it shall be for meat.'

It is only after Man has been expelled from the garden of Eden, that he starts killing for food. Other primitive cultures have essentially similar tales of a fall from a once perfect state of universal kinship. The question is — how do we go about reclaiming Eden?

Change Yourself — Change the World

The act of gathering, preparing and eating food is one of the most fundamental in any form of human society. It is so basic that, much of the time, we forget just how important it is to us, both individually and as a species. It is, in fact, the bedrock that underlies most forms of human economic and political activity. So what happens if we begin to make some pretty basic changes to the way we go about feeding ourselves?

Well, plenty happens. On a personal and purely physical level, you should start to feel in better shape. But that's just the beginning, because the implications of what you're doing will spread far beyond your immediate environment.

At this point, the cynics will tell us that we're foolish to believe such ideas, because the world can't be changed just by one person giving up eating meat. Well, maybe it can't. But it's the *first step*. We have a long way to go, but it is only the first step that is really difficult. If we don't take that first step, the alternative is simply to give up the struggle and abandon our world to the darkness that threatens it. 'In a just cause,' said Sophocles in 401 B.C., 'the weak will beat the strong.'

We Can Change Things for the Better

Let's talk about specifics. Here are just some of the benefits — immediate, real and tangible — that will start to occur as more and more people in this country take control of this crucial area of their lives, and start to kick the flesh food habit.

- We will import far less grain for animal food. Britain *could* be self-sufficient in grain, if we didn't feed so much to our food animals. At the moment, we spend over £4000 million *every year* on importing food and feedstuff from overseas, and we feed our farm animals an amount of grain equivalent to the total amount that we presently grow in this country.
- Diet-related disease will drop dramatically.
- The process of intensification of food production will be reversed, allowing more people to be employed (we won't need to be quite so ruthlessly efficient as we are at the moment, because we will be able to *directly use* vastly more of the food we *do* produce, instead of wasting most of it by feeding it to meat animals).
- A declining market for animal feed and animal flesh will allow developing countries to concentrate on what they *need* to produce for themselves, rather than on what they *have* to produce

for the greedy West (as recently as 1984 Britain was importing over a million pounds worth of animal feed and flesh from — of all places — Ethiopia).

- The world's soya crop (perhaps one of our most under-utilized resources) will begin to be used as it should be — for direct, high-quality human food, and not fed to meat animals as it is at the moment (the EEC alone imports 20 million tons every year just to be fed to animals).

- With more of the energy being put into the process of food production coming from human, rather than fossil-fuel sources, we will be able to use our dwindling natural energy resources in a more productive way.

- Once-effective human medicines will again be able to be used on humans, with far less fear of antibiotic resistance.

- Less official food-price manipulation will be necessary, which at the moment results in the nonsensical surpluses of the EEC. Farmers will be more responsive to real public demands.

- The 'grain prairies' of the main cereal-growing regions will become a thing of the past, as we no longer need to force the land to produce every last grain it can (to try and compensate for the gross inefficiency of the vegetable/animal protein conversion process). More variety of vegetable crops will be grown, in response to consumer demand, and the countryside will be able to return to its pre-factory farming days.

All these things, and more, are within our grasp — if we start *now*.

The Turning Point. . .

The next step is up to you. By changing your own life, you will begin to change the world — not a dramatic change, but a *significant* change. And then what next? I hope — and believe — you may want to take things further. The American philosopher Tom Regan summed this up very clearly when he wrote: 'Merely to content oneself with personal abstention [from animal meat] is to become part of the problem, rather than part of the solution'.[1] In other words, it's not enough to just kick the flesh food habit — once you've found the way for yourself, you also have a duty to spread the word to other people. How can you do this? Here are some ideas for you to consider:

- Think about setting up a 'self-help' group in your locality. Many, many people are interested in the idea of going meat-free, but they don't know where to start. I have been to meetings which have attracted over 200 people! For hints on organization, see the Resource Directory.
- Consider running (or getting your local education authority to organize) classes in meat-free cooking. These can be a lot of fun, very social occasions, and give valuable advice and experience.
- Ask a journalist on your local paper to think about setting up a regular meat-free recipe column.
- Get your local radio station to feature a recipe and/or discussion once a month or so.
- See if other local organizations (Women's Institute, Round Table, etc) would like to organize a 'taste-in'.

There are many other individual ways, too, in which you can be a positive force for change — from just lending a book or two to friends, to going out and addressing public meetings yourself. It all counts, and moves this world one step closer to the next, and most exciting, stage in the human race's history. Good luck!

REFERENCES
1. 'The Case for Animal Rights', Professor Tom Regan, *University of California Press*, 1983.

Appendix I

Using the Nutrition-Checker

The Nutrition-Checker has been specially devized for this book, and it's a special way for you to make sure that you're getting the right nutrition in your diet.

It will allow you to quickly and easily calculate the percentage of your Recommended Daily Allowance (R.D.A.) for a selection of important nutrients in *any* food (not just the ones listed). You only need to know two things to use it:

1) the weight of the food you are going to eat, and

2) the amount of nutrient in *any* weight of the food in question.

Where do you find this information? Well, there are many different sources — such as books on nutrition, magazine articles, and increasingly on food labels themselves. More and more manufacturers are starting to reveal nutritional analyses of their food on the packets, and the Nutrition-Checker will enable you to make sense of it — and relate it to your own *personal* needs.

It's best if you have a calculator handy, as it will enable you to perform the calculation in a matter of a second or two, although you can do it with a paper and pencil if you want. This example shows how it works:

QUESTION: *You've bought a frozen cheese and tomato pizza, and want to find out how much of your day's requirement for protein you will get if you eat half of it. The label says that the whole thing weighs 520 grams, and it contains a total of 62.4 grams of protein. Just for good measure, it also tells you that there are 12 grams of protein in every 100 grams weight of the pizza.*

Well for a start, you don't actually need all this information. You will be able to use Nutrition-Checker with *either* of the two sets of information they've given you.

This is what you do:

Step One

The first thing to do is to calculate the *weight* of the food you're actually going to eat. How do you do this? You could do it in several ways:

- You could actually weigh it in the kitchen — although you might not always have same scales handy.
- Do some mental arithmetic. You know the whole pizza weighs 520 grams — so divide 520 by 2 to find out that half of it will weigh 260 grams. And quarter will weigh 130 grams . . . and so on.

Got it? So switch your calculator on and enter the *weight* of the food *that you actually want to eat*. In this case, you want to eat just half the pizza. So the first figure you enter on your calculator is **260**.

Step Two

Press the divide button (÷) on your calculator and enter the weight of the food that you have information about. You've read on the label that the whole pizza weighs 520 grams. So enter **520**.

Step Three

Now press the 'multiply' button (×) on the calculator, and then enter the amount of nutrient contained *in the weight of the food that you've just entered*. On the pizza label, you've read that it contains a total of 62.4 grams of protein in 520 grams total weight. So enter **62.4**.

Step Four

Now check the Protein Calculator (if you were measuring vitamin A, you'd check the vitamin A calculator, and so on). Look along the top until you find the last column, headed Nutrition-Checker. Follow the column down until you find the correct row for you (for example, row U for a moderately active woman aged 18). We'll call the number you find there your *Personal Factor* (in this example, the figure is 1.82). On your calculator, press the 'multiply' button (*) again and enter your *Personal Factor*. In this example you would enter 1.82.

That's it! The calculation is over. Just press the 'equals' button (=) to find the answer to your question. In this case, you'll see that eating half the pizza will supply you with 56.784 per cent of your Recommended Daily Allowance of protein — over half what you need. It's as easy as that!

You will see that each Calculator table in this book includes a Nutrition-Checker column, which you can use in exactly the same way.

Just a word about measurements. We've used food weights in grams throughout, because it makes the process easier and more accurate. However, you may find some information that is given in ounces and want to convert it into grams so you can use Nutrition-Checker. It's simple — just multiply the figure in ounces by 28.35 on your calculator to find its correct weight in grams.

Also, you will sometimes see the abbreviations 'g', 'mg' and 'mcg'. These stand for 'grams', 'milligrams', and 'micrograms' respectively. One milligram is one thousandth of a gram. One microgram is a thousandth of a milligram (i.e. pretty small!).

$$1g = 1,000mg$$
$$1mg = 1,000mcg$$

Nutrients should always be measured in the following units:

Protein:	g
Calcium:	mg
Iron:	mg
Vitamin A:	mcg (retinol equivalent)
Riboflavin:	mg
Pyridoxine:	mg
Nicotinic Acid:	mg

Protein Caculator

		Age	Min. Protein (g)	Rec. Protein (g)
A	Children	Under 1 year	15	20
B		1 year	19	30
C		2 years	21	35
D		3-4 years	25	40
E		5-6 years	28	45
F		7-8 years	30	53
G	Males	9-11 years	36	63
H		12-14 years	46	70
I		15-17 years	50	75
J	sedentary	18-34 years	45	68
K	mod. active	18-34 years	45	75
L	very active	18-34 years	45	90
M	sedentary	35-64 years	43	65
N	mod. active	35-64 years	43	73
O	very active	35-64 years	43	90
P		65-74 years	39	59
Q		75 & over	38	53
R	Females	9-11 years	35	58
S		12-14 years	44	58
T		15-17 years	40	58
U	mod. active	18-54 years	38	55
V	very active	18-54 years	38	63
W		55-74 years	36	51
X		75 & over	34	48
Y	Pregnant		44	60
Z	Lactating		55	68

	Chickpeas % of R.D.A.	Lentils % of R.D.A.	Tofu % of R.D.A.	Whole Wheat Bread % of R.D.A.
A	100.0%	80.0%	58.5%	52.5%
B	66.7%	53.3%	39.0%	35.0%
C	57.1%	45.7%	33.4%	30.0%
D	50.0%	40.0%	29.3%	26.3%
E	44.4%	35.6%	26.0%	23.3%
F	37.7%	30.2%	22.1%	19.8%
G	31.7%	25.4%	18.6%	16.7%
H	28.6%	22.9%	16.7%	15.0%
I	26.7%	21.3%	15.6%	14.0%

	Chickpeas % of R.D.A.	Lentils % of R.D.A.	Tofu % of R.D.A.	Whole Wheat Bread % of R.D.A.
J	29.4%	23.5%	17.2%	15.4%
K	26.7%	21.3%	15.6%	14.0%
L	22.2%	17.8%	13.0%	11.7%
M	30.8%	24.6%	18.0%	16.2%
N	27.4%	21.9%	16.0%	14.4%
O	22.2%	17.8%	13.0%	11.7%
P	33.9%	27.1%	19.8%	17.8%
Q	37.7%	30.2%	22.1%	19.8%
R	34.5%	27.6%	20.2%	18.1%
S	34.5%	27.6%	20.2%	18.1%
T	34.5%	27.6%	20.2%	18.1%
U	36.4%	29.1%	21.3%	19.1%
V	31.7%	25.4%	18.6%	16.7%
W	39.2%	31.4%	22.9%	20.6%
X	41.7%	33.3%	24.4%	21.9%
Y	33.3%	26.7%	19.5%	17.5%
Z	29.4%	23.5%	17.2%	15.4%

	Pasta % of R.D.A.	Cheddar % of R.D.A.	Nuts % of R.D.A.	Soya Beans % of R.D.A.
A	105.0%	155.0%	190.0%	100.0%
B	70.0%	103.3%	126.7%	66.7%
C	60.0%	88.6%	108.6%	57.1%
D	52.5%	77.5%	95.0%	50.0%
E	46.7%	68.9%	84.4%	44.4%
F	39.6%	58.5%	71.7%	37.7%
G	33.3%	49.2%	60.3%	31.7%
H	30.0%	44.3%	54.3%	28.6%
I	28.0%	41.3%	50.7%	26.7%
J	30.9%	45.6%	55.9%	29.4%
K	28.0%	41.3%	50.7%	26.7%
L	23.3%	34.4%	42.2%	22.2%
M	32.3%	47.7%	58.5%	30.8%
N	28.8%	42.5%	52.1%	27.4%
O	23.3%	34.4%	42.2%	22.2%
P	35.6%	52.5%	64.4%	33.9%
Q	39.6%	58.5%	71.7%	37.7%
R	36.2%	53.4%	65.5%	34.5%
S	36.2%	53.4%	65.5%	34.5%
T	36.2%	53.4%	65.5%	34.5%

	Pasta % of R.D.A.	Cheddar % of R.D.A.	Nuts % of R.D.A.	Soya Beans % of R.D.A.
U	38.2%	56.4%	69.1%	36.4%
V	33.3%	49.2%	60.3%	31.7%
W	41.2%	60.8%	74.5%	39.2%
X	43.8%	64.6%	79.2%	41.7%
Y	35.0%	51.7%	63.3%	33.3%
Z	30.9%	45.6%	55.9%	29.4%

	Bulgur Wheat % of R.D.A.	Skim Milk % of R.D.A.	Soya Milk % of R.D.A.	Nutrition-Checker
A	95.0%	—	37.5%	5.00
B	63.3%	—	25.0%	3.33
C	54.3%	—	21.4%	2.86
D	47.5%	—	18.8%	2.50
E	42.4%	19.6%	16.7%	2.22
F	35.8%	16.6%	14.2%	1.89
G	30.2%	14.0%	11.9%	1.59
H	27.1%	12.6%	10.7%	1.43
I	25.3%	11.7%	10.0%	1.33
J	27.9%	12.9%	11.0%	1.47
K	25.3%	11.7%	10.0%	1.33
L	21.1%	9.8%	8.3%	1.11
M	29.2%	13.5%	11.5%	1.54
N	26.0%	12.1%	10.3%	1.37
O	21.1%	9.8%	8.3%	1.11
P	32.2%	14.9%	12.7%	1.69
Q	35.8%	16.6%	14.2%	1.89
R	32.8%	15.2%	12.9%	1.72
S	32.8%	15.2%	12.9%	1.72
T	32.8%	15.2%	12.9%	1.72
U	34.5%	16.0%	13.6%	1.82
V	30.2%	14.0%	11.9%	1.59
W	37.3%	17.3%	14.7%	1.96
X	39.6%	18.3%	15.6%	2.08
Y	31.7%	14.7%	12.5%	1.67
Z	27.9%	12.9%	11.0%	1.47

Notes

Chickpeas: 1 cup cooked = 130 grams, contains 20 grams protein
Lentils: 1 cup cooked = 200 grams, contains 16 grams protein
Tofu: 1 piece of 150 grams (5 ounces) contains 11.7 grams protein
Whole Wheat Bread: 4 slices = 120 grams, contains 10.5 grams protein

Pasta: 100% whole wheat spaghetti, 1 cup = 160 grams, contains 21 grams protein
Cheddar: 120 grams (4 ounces) contains 31 grams protein
Nuts (Peanuts or Sunflower Seeds): 1 cup = 145 grams contains 38 grams protein
Soya beans: 1 cup (cooked) = 180 grams, contains 20 grams protein
Bulgur Wheat: 1 cup uncooked = 170 grams, contains 19 grams protein
Skim Milk: 1 cup contains 8.8 grams protein
Soya Milk: 1 cup plain unfortified contains 7.5 grams protein

Calcium Calculator

		Age	R.D.A. Calcium (mg)	Skim Milk % of R.D.A.
A	Children	Under 1 year	600	—
B		1 year	500	—
C		2 years	500	—
D		3-4 years	500	—
E		5-6 years	500	60.4%
F		7-8 years	500	60.4%
G	Males	9-11 years	700	43.1%
H		12-14 years	700	43.1%
I		15-17 years	600	50.3%
J	sedentary	18-34 years	500	60.4%
K	mod. active	18-34 years	500	60.4%
L	very active	18-34 years	500	60.4%
M	sedentary	35-64 years	500	60.4%
N	mod. active	35-64 years	500	60.4%
O	very active	35-64 years	500	60.4%
P		65-74 years	500	60.4%
Q		75 & over	500	60.4%
R	Females	9-11 years	700	43.1%
S		12-14 years	700	43.1%
T		15-17 years	600	50.3%
U	mod. active	18-54 years	500	60.4%
V	very active	18-54 years	500	60.4%
W		55-74 years	500	60.4%
X		75 & over	500	60.4%
Y	Pregnant		1200	25.2%
Z	Lactating		1200	25.2%

	Dried Milk % of R.D.A.	Dulse % of R.D.A.	Raisins % of R.D.A.	Almonds % of R.D.A.
A	251.3%*	94.5%	17.0%	55.3%

	Dried Milk % of R.D.A.	Dulse % of R.D.A.	Raisins % of R.D.A.	Almonds % of R.D.A.
B	301.6%*	113.4%	20.4%	66.4%
C	301.6%*	113.4%	20.4%	66.4%
D	301.6%*	113.4%	20.4%	66.4%
E	301.6%	113.4%	20.4%	66.4%
F	301.6%	113.4%	20.4%	66.4%
G	215.4%	81.0%	14.6%	47.4%
H	215.4%	81.0%	14.6%	47.4%
I	251.3%	94.5%	17.0%	55.3%
J	301.6%	113.4%	20.4%	66.4%
K	301.6%	113.4%	20.4%	66.4%
L	301.6%	113.4%	20.4%	66.4%
M	301.6%	113.4%	20.4%	66.4%
N	301.6%	113.4%	20.4%	66.4%
O	301.6%	113.4%	20.4%	66.4%
P	301.6%	113.4%	20.4%	66.4%
Q	301.6%	113.4%	20.4%	66.4%
R	215.4%	81.0%	14.6%	47.4%
S	215.4%	81.0%	14.6%	47.4%
T	251.3%	94.5%	17.0%	55.3%
U	301.6%	113.4%	20.4%	66.4%
V	301.6%	113.4%	20.4%	66.4%
W	301.6%	113.4%	20.4%	66.4%
X	301.6%	113.4%	20.4%	66.4%
Y	125.7%	47.3%	8.5%	27.7%
Z	125.7%	47.3%	8.5%	27.7%

*Only if declared suitable for infant use.

	Chickpeas % of R.D.A.	Spinach % of R.D.A.	Cheddar % of R.D.A.	Broccoli % of R.D.A.	Molasses % of R.D.A.	Nutrition-Checker
A	50.0%	27.8%	113.5%	80.0%	46.7%	0.17
B	60.0%	33.4%	136.2%	96.0%	56.0%	0.20
C	60.0%	33.4%	136.2%	96.0%	56.0%	0.20
D	60.0%	33.4%	136.2%	96.0%	56.0%	0.20
E	60.0%	33.4%	136.2%	96.0%	56.0%	0.20
F	60.0%	33.4%	136.2%	96.0%	56.0%	0.20
G	42.9%	23.9%	96.3%	68.6%	40.0%	0.14
H	42.9%	23.9%	97.3%	68.6%	40.0%	0.14
I	50.0%	27.8%	113.5%	80.0%	46.7%	0.17
J	60.0%	33.4%	136.2%	96.0%	56.0%	0.20
K	60.0%	33.4%	136.2%	96.0%	56.0%	0.20

	Chickpeas % of R.D.A.	Spinach % of R.D.A.	Cheddar % of R.D.A.	Broccoli % of R.D.A.	Molasses % of R.D.A.	Nutrition-Checker
L	60.0%	33.4%	136.2%	96.0%	56.0%	0.20
M	60.0%	33.4%	136.2%	96.0%	56.0%	0.20
N	60.0%	33.4%	136.2%	96.0%	56.0%	0.20
O	60.0%	33.4%	136.2%	96.0%	56.0%	0.20
P	60.0%	33.4%	136.2%	96.0%	56.0%	0.20
Q	60.0%	33.4%	136.2%	96.0%	56.0%	0.20
R	42.9%	23.9%	97.3%	68.6%	40.0%	0.14
S	42.9%	23.9%	97.3%	68.6%	40.0%	0.14
T	50.0%	27.8%	113.5%	80.0%	46.7%	0.17
U	60.0%	33.4%	136.2%	96.0%	56.0%	0.20
V	60.0%	33.4%	136.2%	96.0%	56.0%	0.20
W	60.0%	33.4%	136.2%	96.0%	56.0%	0.20
X	60.0%	33.4%	136.2%	96.0%	56.0%	0.20
Y	25.0%	13.9%	56.8%	40.0%	23.3%	0.08
Z	25.0%	13.9%	56.8%	40.0%	23.3%	0.08

Notes

Skim Milk: 1 cup (245 grams) contains 302mg Calcium
Dried Milk: nonfat, 1 cup (120 grams) contains 1508mg Calcium
Dulse: a seaweed (delicious!) that can be bought dried in most whole food shops,
    100 grams (3 ounces) contains 567mg Calcium (Kombu is even higher)
Raisins: 1 cup (165 grams) contains 102mg Calcium
Almonds: 1 cup (142 grams) contains 332mg Calcium
Chickpeas: 1 cup (200 grams) contains 300mg Calcium
Spinach: 1 cup cooked (180 grams) contains 167mg Calcium
Cheddar: a 3 ounce (85 grams) piece contains 681mg Calcium
Broccoli: 3 stalks (540 grams) cooked contains 480mg Calcium
Molasses: 2 tablespoons (40 grams) contains 280mg Calcium

Iron Calculator

		Age	Rec. Iron (mg)	Boiled Egg % of R.D.A.
A	Children	Under 1 year	6	18.33%
B		1 year	7	15.71%
C		2 years	7	15.71%
D		3-4 years	8	13.75%
E		5-6 years	8	13.75%
F		7-8 years	10	11.00%

		Age	Rec. Iron (mg)	Boiled Egg % of R.D.A.
G	Males	9-11 years	13	8.46%
H		12-14 years	14	7.86%
I		15-17 years	15	7.33%
J	sedentary	18-34 years	10	11.00%
K	mod. active	18-34 years	10	11.00%
L	very active	18-34 years	10	11.00%
M	sedentary	35-64 years	10	11.00%
N	mod. active	35-64 years	10	11.00%
O	very active	35-64 years	10	11.00%
P		65-74 years	10	11.00%
Q		75 & over	10	11.00%
R	Females	9-11 years	13	8.46%
S		12-14 years	14	7.86%
T		15-17 years	15	7.33%
U	mod. active	18-54 years	12	9.17%
V	very active	18-54 years	12	9.17%
W		55-74 years	10	11.00%
X		75 & over	10	11.00%
Y	Pregnant		15	7.33%
Z	Lactating		15	7.33%

	Molasses % of R.D.A.	Chickpeas % of R.D.A.	Lentils % of R.D.A.	Spinach % of R.D.A.
A	106.67%	115.00%	70.00%	66.67%
B	91.43%	98.57%	60.00%	57.14%
C	91.43%	98.57%	60.00%	57.14%
D	80.00%	86.25%	52.50%	50.00%
E	80.00%	86.25%	52.50%	50.00%
F	64.00%	69.00%	42.00%	40.00%
G	49.23%	53.08%	32.31%	30.77%
H	45.71%	49.29%	30.00%	28.57%
I	42.67%	46.00%	28.00%	26.67%
J	64.00%	69.00%	42.00%	40.00%
K	64.00%	69.00%	42.00%	40.00%
L	64.00%	69.00%	42.00%	40.00%
M	64.00%	69.00%	42.00%	40.00%
N	64.00%	69.00%	42.00%	40.00%
O	64.00%	69.00%	42.00%	40.00%
P	64.00%	69.00%	42.00%	40.00%
Q	64.00%	69.00%	42.00%	40.00%

	Molasses % of R.D.A.	Chickpeas % of R.D.A.	Lentils % of R.D.A.	Spinach % of R.D.A.
R	49.23%	53.08%	32.31%	30.77%
S	45.71%	49.29%	30.00%	28.57%
T	42.67%	46.00%	28.00%	26.67%
U	53.33%	57.50%	35.00%	33.33%
V	53.33%	57.50%	35.00%	33.33%
W	64.00%	69.00%	42.00%	40.00%
X	64.00%	69.00%	42.00%	40.00%
Y	42.67%	46.00%	28.00%	26.67%
Z	42.67%	46.00%	28.00%	26.67%

	Millet % of R.D.A.	Soya Milk % of R.D.A.	Tofu % of R.D.A.	Whole Wheat Bread % of R.D.A.	Bulgur Wheat % of R.D.A.	Nutrition-Checker
A	130.00%	30.00%	48.33%	46.67%	105.00%	16.67
B	111.43%	25.71%	41.43%	40.00%	90.00%	14.29
C	111.43%	25.71%	41.43%	40.00%	90.00%	14.29
D	97.50%	22.50%	36.25%	35.00%	78.75%	12.50
E	97.50%	22.50%	36.25%	35.00%	78.75%	12.50
F	78.00%	18.00%	29.00%	28.00%	63.00%	10.00
G	60.00%	13.85%	22.31%	21.54%	48.46%	7.69
H	55.71%	12.86%	20.71%	20.00%	45.00%	7.14
I	52.00%	12.00%	19.33%	18.67%	42.00%	6.67
J	78.00%	18.00%	29.00%	28.00%	63.00%	10.00
K	78.00%	18.00%	29.00%	28.00%	63.00%	10.00
L	78.00%	18.00%	29.00%	28.00%	63.00%	10.00
M	78.00%	18.00%	29.00%	28.00%	63.00%	10.00
N	78.00%	18.00%	29.00%	28.00%	63.00%	10.00
O	78.00%	18.00%	29.00%	28.00%	63.00%	10.00
P	78.00%	18.00%	29.00%	28.00%	63.00%	10.00
Q	78.00%	18.00%	29.00%	28.00%	63.00%	10.00
R	60.00%	13.85%	22.31%	21.54%	48.46%	7.69
S	55.71%	12.86%	20.71%	20.00%	45.00%	7.14
T	52.00%	12.00%	19.33%	18.67%	42.00%	6.67
U	65.00%	15.00%	24.17%	23.33%	52.50%	8.33
V	65.00%	15.00%	24.17%	23.33%	52.50%	8.33
W	78.00%	18.00%	29.00%	28.00%	63.00%	10.00
X	78.00%	18.00%	29.00%	28.00%	63.00%	10.00
Y	52.00%	12.00%	19.33%	18.67%	42.00%	6.67
Z	52.00%	12.00%	19.33%	18.67%	42.00%	6.67

Notes

Boiled Egg: one (50 grams) contains 1.1mg Iron

Molasses: 2 tablespoons (40 grams) contains 6.4mg Iron

Chickpeas: 1 cup cooked (100 grams) contains 6.9mg Iron

Lentils: 1 cup cooked (200 grams) contains 4.2mg Iron

Spinach: 1 cup cooked (180 grams) contains 4mg Iron

Millet: half cup dry (114 grams) contains 7.8 grams Iron

Soya Milk: 1 cup plain unfortified contains 1.8mg Iron

Tofu: 1 piece of 150 grams (5 ounces) contains 2.9mg Iron

Whole Wheat Bread: 4 slices (120 grams) contains 2.8mg Iron

Bulgur Wheat: 1 cup uncooked (170 grams) contains, 6.3mg Iron

Vitamin A Calculator

		Age	Rec. Vitamin A (mcg retinol equiv)	Cheddar % of R.D.A.
A	Children	Under 1 year	450	109.78%
B		1 year	300	164.67%
C		2 years	300	164.67%
D		3-4 years	300	164.67%
E		5-6 years	300	164.67%
F		7-8 years	400	123.50%
G	Males	9-11 years	575	85.91%
H		12-14 years	725	68.14%
I		15-17 years	750	65.87%
J	sedentary	18-34 years	750	65.87%
K	mod. active	18-34 years	750	65.87%
L	very active	18-34 years	750	65.87%
M	sedentary	35-64 years	750	65.87%
N	mod. active	35-64 years	750	65.87%
O	very active	35-64 years	750	65.87%
P		65-74 years	750	65.87%
Q		75 & over	750	65.87%
R	Females	9-11 years	575	85.91%
S		12-14 years	725	68.14%
T		15-17 years	750	65.87%
U	mod. active	18-54 years	750	65.87%
V	very active	18-54 years	750	65.87%
W		55-74 years	750	65.87%
X		75 & over	750	65.87%
Y	Pregnant		750	65.87%
Z	Lactating		1200	41.17%

	Carrots % of R.D.A.	Spinach % of R.D.A.	Broccoli % of R.D.A.	Nori % of R.D.A.
A	350.00%	333.33%	300.00%	207.78%
B	525.00%	500.00%	450.00%	311.67%
C	525.00%	500.00%	450.00%	311.67%
D	525.00%	500.00%	450.00%	311.67%
E	525.00%	500.00%	450.00%	311.67%
F	393.75%	375.00%	337.50%	233.75%
G	273.91%	260.87%	234.78%	162.61%
H	217.24%	206.90%	186.21%	128.97%
I	210.00%	200.00%	180.00%	124.67%
J	210.00%	200.00%	180.00%	124.67%
K	210.00%	200.00%	180.00%	124.67%
L	210.00%	200.00%	180.00%	124.67%
M	210.00%	200.00%	180.00%	124.67%
N	210.00%	200.00%	180.00%	124.67%
O	210.00%	200.00%	180.00%	124.67%
P	210.00%	200.00%	180.00%	124.67%
Q	210.00%	200.00%	180.00%	124.67%
R	273.91%	260.87%	234.78%	162.61%
S	217.24%	206.90%	186.21%	128.97%
T	210.00%	200.00%	180.00%	124.67%
U	210.00%	200.00%	180.00%	124.67%
V	210.00%	200.00%	180.00%	124.67%
W	210.00%	200.00%	180.00%	124.67%
X	210.00%	200.00%	180.00%	124.67%
Y	210.00%	200.00%	180.00%	124.67%
Z	131.25%	125.00%	112.50%	77.92%

	Dried Apricots % of R.D.A.	Mango % of R.D.A.	Peach % of R.D.A.	Prunes % of R.D.A.	Red Pepper % of R.D.A.	Nutrition- Checker
A	314.89%	246.44%	29.56%	35.33%	98.89%	0.22
B	472.33%	369.67%	44.33%	53.00%	148.33%	0.33
C	472.33%	369.67%	44.33%	53.00%	148.33%	0.33
D	472.33%	369.67%	44.33%	53.00%	148.33%	0.33
E	472.33%	369.67%	44.33%	53.00%	148.33%	0.33
F	354.25%	277.25%	33.25%	39.75%	111.25%	0.25
G	246.43%	192.87%	23.13%	27.65%	77.39%	0.17
H	195.45%	152.97%	18.34%	21.93%	61.38%	0.14
I	188.93%	147.87%	17.73%	21.20%	59.33%	0.13
J	188.93%	147.87%	17.73%	21.20%	59.33%	0.13
K	188.93%	147.87%	17.73%	21.20%	59.33%	0.13

	Dried Apricots % of R.D.A.	Mango % of R.D.A.	Peach % of R.D.A.	Prunes % of R.D.A.	Red Pepper % of R.D.A.	Nutrition-Checker
L	188.93%	147.87%	17.73%	21.20%	59.33%	0.13
M	188.93%	147.87%	17.73%	21.20%	59.33%	0.13
N	188.93%	147.87%	17.73%	21.20%	59.33%	0.13
O	188.93%	147.87%	17.73%	21.20%	59.33%	0.13
P	188.93%	147.87%	17.73%	21.20%	59.33%	0.13
Q	188.93%	147.87%	17.73%	21.20%	59.33%	0.13
R	246.43%	192.87%	23.13%	27.65%	77.39%	0.17
S	195.45%	152.97%	18.34%	21.93%	61.38%	0.14
T	188.93%	147.87%	17.73%	21.20%	59.33%	0.13
U	188.93%	147.87%	17.73%	21.20%	59.33%	0.13
V	188.93%	147.87%	17.73%	21.20%	59.33%	0.13
W	188.93%	147.87%	17.73%	21.20%	59.33%	0.13
X	188.93%	147.87%	17.73%	21.20%	59.33%	0.13
Y	188.93%	147.87%	17.73%	21.20%	59.33%	0.13
Z	118.08%	92.42%	11.08%	13.25%	37.08%	0.08

Notes

Cheddar: 120 grams (4 ounces) contains 494mcg Vitamin A (retinol equivalent)

Carrots: 1 cup cooked (155grams) contains 1575mcg Vitamin A (retinol equivalent)

Spinach: 1 cup cooked (180 grams) contains 1500mcg Vitamin A (retinol equivalent)

Broccoli: 3 stalks (540 grams) contains 1350mcg Vitamin A (retinol equivalent)

Nori (a seaweed): 85 grams (3 ounces) contains 935mcg Vitamin A (retinol equivalent)

Dried Apricots: 1 cup (130 grams) contains 1417mcg Vitamin A (retinol equivalent)

Mango (raw): 1 average (300 grams) contains 1109mcg Vitamin A (retinol equivalent)

Peach: 1 average (115 grams) contains 133mcg Vitamin A (retinol equivalent)

Prunes: 1 cup cooked (250 grams) contains 159mcg Vitamin A (retinol equivalent)

Red Pepper (not the hot kind): 1 cup sliced raw (100) contains 445mcg Vitamin A (retinol equivalent)

Riboflavin Calculator

	Age	Rec. Riboflavin (mg)	Cheddar % of R.D.A.
A	Children	Under 1 year 0.4	150.00%
B		1 year 0.6	100.00%
C		2 years 0.7	85.71%
D		3-4 years 0.8	75.00%

		Age	Rec. Riboflavin (mg)	Cheddar % of R.D.A.
E		5-6 years	0.9	66.67%
F		7-8 years	1	60.00%
G	Males	9-11 years	1.2	50.00%
H		12-14 years	1.4	42.86%
I		15-17 years	1.7	35.29%
J	sedentary	18-34 years	1.7	35.29%
K	mod. active	18-34 years	1.7	35.29%
L	very active	18-34 years	1.7	35.29%
M	sedentary	35-64 years	1.7	35.29%
N	mod. active	35-64 years	1.7	35.29%
O	very active	35-64 years	1.7	35.29%
P		65-74 years	1.7	35.29%
Q		75 & over	1.7	35.29%
R	Females	9-11 years	1.2	50.00%
S		12-14 years	1.4	42.86%
T		15-17 years	1.4	42.86%
U	mod. active	18-54 years	1.3	46.15%
V	very active	18-54 years	1.3	46.15%
W		55-74 years	1.3	46.15%
X		75 & over	1.3	46.15%
Y	Pregnant		1.6	37.50%
Z	Lactating		1.8	33.33%

	Broccoli % of R.D.A.	Almonds % of R.D.A.	Spinach % of R.D.A.	Skim Milk % of R.D.A.
A	270.00%	325.00%	62.50%	—
B	180.00%	216.67%	41.67%	—
C	154.29%	185.71%	35.71%	—
D	135.00%	162.50%	31.25%	—
E	120.00%	144.44%	27.78%	48.89%
F	108.00%	130.00%	25.00%	44.00%
G	90.00%	108.33%	20.83%	36.67%
H	77.14%	92.86%	17.86%	31.43%
I	63.53%	76.47%	14.71%	25.88%
J	63.53%	76.47%	14.71%	25.88%
K	63.53%	76.47%	14.71%	25.88%
L	63.53%	75.47%	14.71%	25.88%
M	63.53%	76.47%	14.71%	25.88%
N	63.53%	76.47%	14.71%	25.88%

	Broccoli % of R.D.A.	Almonds % of R.D.A.	Spinach % of R.D.A.	Skim Milk % of R.D.A.
O	63.53%	76.47%	14.71%	25.88%
P	63.53%	76.47%	14.71%	25.88%
Q	63.53%	76.47%	14.71%	25.88%
R	90.00%	108.33%	20.83%	36.67%
S	77.14%	92.86%	17.86%	31.43%
T	77.14%	92.86%	17.86%	31.43%
U	83.08%	100.00%	19.23%	33.85%
V	83.08%	100.00%	19.23%	33.85%
W	83.08%	100.00%	19.23%	33.85%
X	83.08%	100.00%	19.23%	33.85%
Y	67.50%	81.25%	15.63%	27.50%
Z	60.00%	72.22%	13.89%	24.44%

	Millet % of R.D.A.	Avocado % of R.D.A.	Chickpeas % of R.D.A.	Brewers Yeast % of R.D.A.	Yeast Extract % of R.D.A.	Nutrition-Checker
A	110.00%	100.00%	32.50%	85.00%	220.00%	250.00
B	73.33%	66.67%	21.67%	56.67%	146.67%	166.67
C	62.86%	57.14%	18.57%	48.57%	125.71%	142.86
D	55.00%	50.00%	16.25%	42.50%	110.00%	125.00
E	48.89%	44.44%	14.44%	37.78%	97.78%	111.11
F	44.00%	40.00%	13.00%	34.00%	88.00%	100.00
G	36.67%	33.33%	10.83%	28.33%	73.33%	83.33
H	31.43%	28.57%	9.29%	24.29%	62.86%	71.43
I	25.88%	23.53%	7.65%	20.00%	51.76%	58.82
J	25.88%	23.53%	7.65%	20.00%	51.76%	58.82
K	25.88%	23.52%	7.65%	20.00%	51.76%	58.82
L	25.88%	23.53%	7.65%	20.00%	51.76%	58.82
M	25.88%	23.53%	7.65%	20.00%	51.76%	58.82
N	25.88%	23.53%	7.65%	20.00%	51.76%	58.82
O	25.88%	23.53%	7.65%	20.00%	51.76%	58.82
P	25.88%	23.53%	7.65%	20.00%	51.76%	58.82
Q	25.88%	23.53%	7.65%	20.00%	51.76%	58.82
R	36.67%	33.33%	10.83%	28.33%	73.33%	83.33
S	31.43%	28.57%	9.29%	24.29%	62.86%	71.43
T	31.43%	28.57%	9.29%	24.29%	62.86%	71.43
U	33.85%	30.77%	10.00%	26.15%	67.69%	76.92
V	33.85%	30.77%	10.00%	26.15%	67.69%	76.92
W	33.85%	30.77%	10.00%	26.15%	67.69%	76.92
X	33.85%	30.77%	10.00%	26.15%	67.69%	76.92
Y	27.50%	25.00%	8.13%	21.25%	55.00%	62.50
Z	24.44%	22.22%	7.22%	18.89%	48.89%	55.56

Notes

Cheddar: 120 grams (4 ounces) contains 0.6mg riboflavin
Broccoli: 3 stalks (540 grams) contains 1.08mg riboflavin
Almonds: 1 cup (142 grams) contains 1.3mg riboflavin
Spinach: 1 cup cooked (180 grams) contains 0.25mg riboflavin
Skim Milk: 1 cup (245 grams) contains 0.4mg riboflavin
Millet: half cup dry (114 grams) contains 0.44 riboflavin
Avocado: 1 average (200 grams without stone) contains 0.4mg riboflavin
Chickpeas: 1 cup (200 grams) contains 0.13mg riboflavin
Brewers Yeast: 1 tablespoon (8 grams) contains 0.34mg riboflavin
Yeast Extract: 1 tablespoon (8 grams) contains 0.88mg riboflavin

Pyridoxine Calculator

		R.D.A. (mg)	Nutri-Check
Children	0-6 months	0.3	333.33
	7-11 months	0.4	250.00
	1-3 years	0.8	125.00
	4-6 years	1.3	76.92
Males	7-9 years	1.6	62.50
	10-12 years	1.8	55.56
	13 and over	2	50.00
Females	7-9 years	1.4	71.43
	10 and over	1.5	66.67
	Pregnant	add 0.5	50.00
	Lactating	add 0.6	47.62

Appendix II

Resource Directory

Agar-Agar
A vegetable equivalent of gelatine, made from seaweed, a good source of minerals, and available at most wholefood shops.

Chickpeas
A very ancient food from the Near East, India and many other warm countries, found cultivated in the Hanging Gardens of Babylon, and mentioned in the Bible. Don't buy tinned chickpeas, they're expensive and not nearly so tasty. Dried chickpeas will store very well, and will reconstitute after overnight soaking and pressure cooking. They can be used to make falafel, hummus and delicious soups, and they are wonderful cold in salads. When ground they are called Gram Flour (or Besan) used in much Indian cuisine (called Channa), including onion bajis.

Dieting and Losing Weight
Don't bother about trying to lose weight if you've recently gone meat-free, you may find that your body will naturally stabilize at an optimum weight, and it's more difficult to over-eat without all those saturated fat calories in meat. If you then want to diet, here's a tip. Try a mainly raw food diet, it's almost impossible to over-eat on raw food. *Don't* go on crash diets, they don't work, and may jeopardize your health. Cut out junk food *first*. Physical activity is important too, not because it burns up lots of calories (it doesn't), but because your body's mechanisms will tend to regulate your

appetite to match your new activity level. If you have diabetes or other metabolic diseases, or are pregnant, *don't* diet without consulting your doctor. Forget about the fad and 'latest craze' diets, there's only one way you're going to lose weight, and that's by restricting your total calorie intake, and increasing your calorie expenditure.

Dogs and Cats
Dogs and cats that are fed exclusively on meat have been found to develop soft bones and become in generally poor condition. On the other hand, however, cats cannot metabolize certain nutrients from vegetable sources, and so you need to include some scraps from the fishmonger in their diet on a regular basis. Otherwise, the easiest way to feed dogs and cats is simply to include them when preparing human food.

Eggs
In this country, we have some genuinely humane legislation entitled the Protection of Birds Act 1954, which says:
'If any person keeps or confines any bird whatsoever in any cage or other receptacle which is not sufficient in height, length or breadth to permit the bird to stretch its wings freely, he shall be guilty of an offence against the Act and be liable to a special penalty.'
Which sounds all very well and good, until you read the next clause that was inserted into the Act before it became law:
'Provided that this subsection shall not apply to poultry.'
Of course this makes the Act a complete travesty, and testifies to the parliamentary influence of the food industry. There is no doubt that battery hens lead utterly horrifying lives, as anyone who has visited a battery unit must agree. The alternative is free range, and is becoming very much more popular all the time. You can do your bit, by only buying free-range eggs. Further information: Compassion in World Farming (for address see 'Films'), or Chickens Lib, 6 Pilling Lane, Skelmanthorpe, Huddersfield, West Yorks, telephone 0484-861814 or Free-Range Egg Association, 37 Tanza Road, London NW3 5SG, telephone 01-435 2596.

Elderly, Special Needs of

Old people can thrive on a meat-free diet, and many report that cutting meat out actually improves their bodily health and sense of vigour. The elderly no longer need to grow, so don't need quite so much carbohydrates, fats or proteins, but still have a great requirement for good quality vitamins and minerals. A food processor will prove useful to chop fresh food into easy size pieces, and will make delicious and nourishing soups and purees. Both fresh and dried fruit have a useful place in each day's diet. Many older people prefer smaller amounts of food at more frequent intervals. Regular exercise, sunshine, pure water and good companionship are essential too.

Films, for Public Exhibition

A number of organizations have films and videos for hire, often at no or low cost. Concord Films Council, 201 Felixstowe Road, Ipswich, Suffolk, IP3 9BJ, telephone 0473 76012 have a very good catalogue (sae for current price list) which includes the impressive *Vegetarian World* presented by William Shatner (Captain Kirk from TV's *Star Trek*). Other organizations having films for hire include: RSPCA, Causeway, Horsham, Sussex RH12 1HG, telephone 0403-64181; BBC Enterprises Educational Sales, Woodlands, 80 Wood Lane, London W12 0TT, telephone 01-576 0202; Compassion in World Farming, 20 Lavant Street, Petersfield, Hants GU32 3EW, telephone 0730-64208.

Group, Organizing a

An informally organized self-help group, operating in your local community, is by far the best way of taking things a stage further. If you are worried that you don't know enough to organise such a group, then you're probably *exactly* the right person to do it! All you need to start with is one or two more like-minded people to yourself. To find them, try putting up a card or poster in suitable locations (wholefood shops, restaurants, etc), saying something like: 'Giving Meat the Chop? Self-help group starting for people who want to spread the word about meat-free cooking and living. Needs help and ideas from people like you . . . Contact me for a chat: (your name and 'phone number/address)'. Then fix a date for the first planning meeting (possibly held at your house). Make the meeting very informal. Everyone must have the chance to express themselves. Don't vote on anything — come to an agreed consensus instead. You may have to lead the discussion, but *don't dictate!* These are some suggestions for the areas you should aim to discuss.

- The name of the group (have at least three suggestions ready).
- Its objects (suggestion: to convert more people in your area to meat-free living).
- Activities (suggestions — four large public events a year; four issues of a magazine a year; cookery demonstrations, special restaurant evenings, all-day food fairs with stands for other organizations, leafletting).
- Who is going to be responsible for certain areas (e.g. finance, chairperson, publicity, secretary).

The real key to success is publicity, and that means hard work for everyone. Draw up a 'Contact List' together, with all the people who need to be notified in advance of your events (TV, radio, press) and all the places where you can display posters (aim to get at least fifty posters out four weeks before any event, in all libraries, shops, large businesses, public buildings, etc). Street leafletting a day or two before the event is very worthwhile, too, if you can get several thousand handbills cheaply produced. There is a lot of satisfaction in helping to run a self-help group, and it could open new horizons for you.

Herbs and Spices
Nothing looks nicer than a kitchen lined with glass jars full of intriguing herbs and spices. Experiment and build up your collection as you go along, it's the only way to learn. Avoid commercial concoctions (e.g. garam masala) and grind your own instead, they will taste infinitely better, and you can suit them to your own palate. Buy small quantities as a rule, since they can deteriorate with time. Just a few particularly useful ones:

- Basil or Oregano — Either of these are especially exciting when added to tomato in dishes such as Tomato Soup, Vegetable

Lasagna, Tomato Salad, etc. Only a little is needed when the herb is cooked.

- Chives — You can purchase these dried, but they are also fun and easy to grow. Use them in salads, soups, sandwiches and flans for their bright colour and subtle onion flavour.
- Cumin — Buy this spice whole and grind it yourself when you need it. At its best in rice or lentil dishes, a rather strong flavour adding depth to the dish.
- Ginger — Most people know what this tastes like, but did you know that it may be used fresh or dried in soups, salads, curries, beverages and a dozen other dishes without ever seeming the same? You can pickle fresh ginger in sherry to keep well (store it in the fridge).
- Mint — Use it fresh in season and dry all the winter to liven up beverages, salads and their dressings, or to enhance peas, potatoes and pasta. Experiment with the different types of mint to find your favourite, e.g. spearmint, applemint, peppermint.
- Mustard — That's the seed (black or yellow) or the dry mustard powder (which is ground yellow mustard seed). Use mustard seed in dressings, stir-fries or curries. Use the powder in dressings or sauces but use a light hand to start with.
- Paprika — Part of the chilli family but not so hot. Paprika is full of vitamins A and C, goes well in cheese dishes, salads and dressings. A sprinkle of it before serving ensures that none of its value is lost.
- Parsley — This herb may be used dried in soups, stews, salads or baked dishes. Fresh, it is often used as a garnish: be sure to eat it as it is high in vitamins A and C. It has a strong flavour, but one which clears your taste-buds for the next dish.
- Sage — Use this herb sparingly as its flavour is both strong and distinctive. It is used in stuffings, nut dishes, sauces and combined with other herbs in stews or casseroles.
- Tarragon — Another distinct flavour, but this time more subtle. Tarragon may be used fresh or dried in egg dishes, salads and their dressings, sauces and herb butters and with leafy vegetables and avocados.

- Thyme — At its best with foods that are to some extent fatty, such as beans, cheeses, dressings, sauces and marinades; or sprinkle a pinch of fresh or dried thyme over a tomato salad. This herb helps digestion.

Lentils

A leguminous plant, popular with Homo Sapiens since the Bronze Age, whose seeds are twenty-five per cent protein, rich in B vitamins, iron and phosphorus. There are many different colours and varieties, and they feature in Indian and Middle Eastern cuisine. You must cook them thoroughly (soft, not crunchy to the palate). If you still get a tummy upset after having eaten them, it may be because the intestinal flora of your stomach is changing to accomodate your new diet, and things will get better after a week or two. You may have to keep a watchful eye on them as you pour them out, before rinsing, as small stones sometimes get mixed up with them! There are literally hundreds of ways of presenting them in creative cuisine. As with all beans and pulses they're much cheaper if you can buy a sackful at a time.

Miso

Fermented soya bean paste, an essential for Japanese and Chinese cooking. High protein, low calorie, many different varieties, substitute for salt in most recipes.

Organic Food

A third of the fruit and vegetables on sale in this country contains detectable traces of pesticide residue, according to a recent survey, including such notorious compounds as DDT. There are no legal limits on pesticide residues, so it's a case of the buyer having to beware. You can avoid this problem by buying (or better still, growing) organic fruit and vegetables. Also, you won't believe how different they taste — it's a real revelation! Information on organic gardening from the Henry Doubleday Research Association, Ryton on Dunsmore, Coventry, or from The Soil Association Ltd, Walnut Tree Manor, Haughley, Stowmarket, Suffolk IP14 3RS, telephone 0449-673235; or from the Good Gardeners Association, CRG

Shewell-Cooper, Arkley Manor Farm, Rowley Lane, Arkley, Barnet, Herts EN5 3HS, telephone 01-449 7944, who also run training courses with diplomas.

Organizations, Joining

There are a very few organizations that represent the interests of people who don't eat meat. I can't honestly recommend that you join any of them, unless you do so specifically because you want to change them in some way. They tend to be very old-fashioned and unrepresentative in their attitudes, and it is debatable whether they achieve very much more than being a warm place for their committee members to meet each other. Turnover of new members tends to be high, possibly because they don't find the help they're looking for. A much more constructive idea is to start your own self-help group locally — you'll do more good, and have very much more fun! *See* Group, Organizing a.

Rennet (in Cheese)

An enzyme taken from the stomachs of slaughtered baby calfs, a very small amount of which helps to coagulate milk into cheese. Not all cheese includes animal rennet by any means, but if you want to be sure, buy a specially-marked cheese from a health food shop, or a growing number of supermarkets.

Restaurants/Setting up in Business

If you find the idea of starting your own restaurant or wholefood business attractive, you should remember that both these activities involve extremely hard work, often for little or no reward, and major risk to your own capital. Someone once said that there are just three important things to consider when setting up a restaurant — location, location and location. But to secure the best locations, you may have to pay dearly. Which means that you have to be sure of having a sizeable number of customers. It is essential to do some budgets early on, or you may otherwise find that you cannot possibly make any money, no matter how hard you work. The Hotel and Catering Industry Training Board runs introductory courses, P.O. Box 18, Ramsey House, Central Square, Wembley HA9 67AP, telephone 01-902 8865. If you're planning a co-operative venture, contact the National Co-Operative Development Agency Broadmead House, 21 Panton Street, London SW1Y 4DR, telephone 01-839 2985, and ask at your local town hall as well. Your local Small Firms Information Service may be able to help as well, dial the operator and ask for Freephone 2444. Other organisations of possible interest include: National Association of Shopkeepers, Lynch House, 91 Mansfield Road, Nottingham NG1 3FN, telephone 0602-475046; Manpower Services Commission Enterprise Allowance Scheme contact your local Job Centre for current details. If you have a friendly bank manager use him for all he (or she) is worth as a source of up to date information. And don't take no for an answer — from anyone!

Rice

The staple food of more than two billion people on this planet, and a superior food not likely to cause allergy. Avoid white or polished rice, which has had most of the goodness (B vitamins, fat and protein) destroyed during processing. Rice flour contains no gluten and can be used for puddings, pastries and cakes, but not bread. Wild rice is a totally different plant.

Seaweed

The thought of cooking with seaweed may fill you with horror, but if so, think again. For a start, try Kombu (Kelp), a single strip of which can simply be added to any soup or stew you're making, at the beginning of cooking. Leave it in the pot, and it will thicken and bring out the flavour of whatever else you put in. You'll be amazed how you can make a delicious soup from nothing other than kombu, water and vegetables. When you've found your sea-legs, try experimenting with Nori, Arame, and Dulse.

Sprouting

A do-it-yourself home garden which, for a few pence, will provide you with an unrivalled source of fresh nutritious vegetables all year round, while boosting your vitamin C intake. You can sprout mung beans (the usual sort of bean sprouts) and also chickpeas, lentils, fenugreek, alfalfa, mustard seeds, etc. Wash the seeds, soak in cold water overnight. Then drain, place in jar, cover the top with cloth and secure with a rubber band, and through this rinse the beans twice a day, draining each time. In a day or two you'll have perfect bean sprouts. Don't let them stand in water, or they'll rot. Don't, whatever you do, use seeds intended for agricultural use, as their dressing may be poisonous.

Tahini
A paste made from ground sesame seeds and oil, very high in calcium if it's made with brown unhulled sesame seeds. Very tasty when used in recipes, an ingredient of hummus, and will often serve as an egg substitute in many dishes.

Tamari (or Shoyu or Soya Sauce)
Throw out the supermarket soya sauce, it's made with hydrochloric acid and is nothing like the original. Buy instead shoyu, which is brewed for four to six months from defatted soya meal, or tamari, which is more expensive and traditionally Japanese, fermented for twelve or eighteen months. You'll notice the difference.

Tempeh
A traditional Japanese fermented soya product, available in many wholefood shops, very high in usable protein and a source of vitamin B^{12}. More difficult to make at home than tofu, since it needs fermenting with a special mycelium *Rhizopus*.

Tofu
Soya bean curd that can be bought in wholefood shops or easily made at home. Very high in protein, extremely adaptable in recipes, low in fat. Some books suggest making it from soya flour, but don't, as it will be gritty. Can be made either runny (for dressings etc.) or firm (for frying) depending on the curdling agent (lemon juice, cider vinegar or the original *nigari*, again available from wholefood shops). Many books now show you the simple process, the easiest description being in *The Farm Vegetarian Cookbook*. Will freeze for months.

Travelling, Eating on the Run
The facilities in this country for good, healthy eating while travelling are almost always horrific in the extreme. Neither the caterers at

motorway service areas, nor the chefs at British Rail, seem to have heard about the coronary heart disease epidemic. There are just three things we can do: 1) campaign vociferously for better quality food; 2) using guides and local information try to track down a few good restaurants; 3) pack your own travelling snacks.

Utensils

No gadgets, here are a few beneficial tools for your kitchen:

- Pressure cooker (a must for beans and pulses).
- Cast-iron pans (or enamel, but no aluminium or copper).
- Wok (for really fast stir-frying of vegetables using minimal oil or, with care, can even be used without any oil if you watch over it and sprinkle water on when necessary).
- Garlic press (releases the flavour better than chopping).
- Mouli (more effort than an electric blender, but cheaper).
- Grater (more effort than a food processor, but much cheaper, and allows you to eat such delicious raw salad vegetables as beetroot, turnip, swede, carrot, etc).
- Steamer (never boil the nutrients in vegetables away again!).
- Mortar and pestle (for grinding spices).

Vegetarian

An old-fashioned name for someone who doesn't eat meat.

Yogurt

This 'live' food maintains or introduces to your intestines bacteria that are necessary for healthy digestion but also helpful in preventing harmful bacteria from establishing. Yogurt is high in protein and the B-group of vitamins and is known to have more of vitamins A and D than the milk from which it was made. It is recommended for persons with lactose intolerance as well as those who have recently taken a course of antibiotics (which destroy beneficial bacteria in the intestines). Babies and young children thrive on fresh yogurt as it resembles human milk and is therefore unlikely to cause allergy. Any milk may be used to make yogurt and this explains its presence all around the world. It is a versatile food and one that is easily made following a simple procedure:

Sterilize a jar or container with boiling water — include the lids and any spoons you will use to stir the yogurt. Decide which milk you wish to use i.e. soya, whole or skimmed cow's milk. Measure 1 litre (approx. 2 pints) of the milk into a saucepan and place it over a medium heat. If using cow's milk, heat the milk until it begins to break into small bubbles at the edges of the pan. If using soya milk, actually boil the milk for 30-60 seconds (be sure you keep stirring). Remove the milk from the heat and pour it into the containers you have sterilized. Cover the containers with their lids or a clean cloth and allow the milk to cool to just warmer than blood heat (if splashed onto your wrist it should feel warm but not hot). Now stir in two rounded dessertspoons of purchased plain, live, unsweetened yogurt with a sterilized spoon. Cover the containers with their lids. Place the containers where they will be kept a constant temperature of 44°C/100°F for 2-6 hours. An airing cupboard, the top of a refrigerator or near the pilot light on a cooker will do nicely. Wrap the container in a tea cosy or towel to ensure the temperature is kept. The yogurt will become thicker the longer you leave it warming, i.e. over-night. Store the yogurt in the refrigerator and keep a small amount separate for the 'starter' to your next batch.

Britain Challenges European Ban
on Hormone Growth Promoters

On 10 March 1986 Britain's Minister of Agriculture, Michael Jopling, made this statement to Parliament:

The Government has today made an application to the European Court of Justice seeking annulment of the EEC Directive banning the use of hormone growth promoters. This action reflects our objections to the basis upon which this Directive was adopted, including the lack of regard for relevant scientific evidence. In taking this action in the European Court, the Government does not seek to discourage producers who wish to rear animals without the use of added hormones. Until a ban is implemented, this remains a matter for commercial decision of individual farmers.

Index

An Invitation to Contribute to Future Editions

The author would welcome contributions from readers for future updated and enlarged editions of this book, particularly from people who work in the meat, food or agricultural industries. Strict anonymity will be respected where requested. Please write to: Peter Cox, 'Why You Don't Need Meat', Thorsons Publishing Group Ltd, Denington Estate, Wellingborough, Northants, NN8 2RQ.

The Vegetarian Cookbook

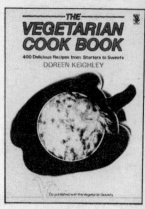

Doreen Keighley presents the greatest variety of vegetarian meals you are ever likely to find anywhere. Covers everything from Brazil nut and tomato roast to digestive biscuits. *All recipes thoroughly tested and produced in conjunction with the Vegetarian Society of the United Kingdom.*

Let's Cook It Together

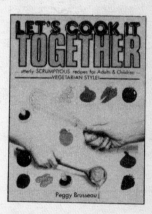

Utterly Scrumptious Recipes for Adults and Children — Vegetarian Style

Peggy Brusseau. This unique cookery book presents over 100 original recipes in a clear step-by-step format for parents and children to use together. Uses symbols to show who does what.